Praise for *Ask Dr. Nandi*

Ask Dr. Nandi and #HealthHeroes are brilliant brands for today—a time when "high touch" is needed even more than "high tech." Partha Nandi is going to impact more people's lives with his platform than anyone prior and I am thrilled to see that.

Nan-Kirsten Forte, MS, WebMD pioneer and
SVP Brand Marketing, Healthline

Dr. Nandi is a celebrated medical doctor and colleague who has a blueprint for health that offers no doctor visits, tests, or pills. The plan has five simple steps that together add power, strength, and purpose to our lives. As Dr. Nandi says, "if you want to do better, you must first know better," *Ask Dr. Nandi* is the key to a healthy kingdom where stress does not corrode your life, where bonds are strong, and the food is clean and nourishing. A must-read for you and your family"

Joel K. Kahn, MD, FACC, Professor of Medicine and
author of *The Whole Heart Solution*

Dr. Nandi's new book, *Ask Dr. Nandi: 5 Steps to Becoming Your Own #HealthHero for Longevity, Well-Being, and a Joyful Life* is a lively, informative, and practical owners manual for living a joyful life, fueled by purpose. Partha is a dedicated physician as well an engaging storyteller, and his book is his gift to humanity. His message is as profound as it is simple: treat your body like it belongs to someone you love, and with the right mind-set, you can fulfill your greatest dreams.

Pankaj Vij, MD, FACP, author of *Turbo Metabolism:*
12 Steps to a New You: Preventing and Reversing Diabetes
and Other Metabolic Diseases by Treating the Causes

Dr. Nandi walks through the five key pillars that we need for happy, long lives. Instead of focusing on one disease or ailment, Dr. Nandi gives us a total, holistic prescription to live to our fullest potentials. *Ask Dr. Nandi* is powerful for two reasons. First, his advice about finding and cultivating your tribe is compelling. Too often, the connection with other people in our communities is lost today in our busy, online world. Second, Dr. Nandi offers simple techniques to become more mindful and incorporate meditation into our daily lives. Guided by this book, anyone can live a more joyful, health-minded lifestyle.

Mark Hyman, MD, Director of the Cleveland
Clinic Center for Functional Medicine

Dr. Partha reaches more than eighty million people daily with his wildly popular television show, *Ask Dr. Nandi*, and now you can bring his powerful advice home with his book. He outlines his simple yet comprehensive plan to uplevel your health and your life. Learn why millions rely on Dr. Nandi daily for their health.

JJ Virgin, CNS, CHFS, nutrition and fitness expert and
New York Times bestselling author of *The Virgin Diet*,
Sugar Impact Diet, and *Miracle Mindset*

Ask Dr. Nandi is a simple, thought-provoking plan that will bring the best practices for healthy living into your home. Dr. Nandi and his family have dedicated themselves to teaching us how to stay out of the doctor's office with simple, doable lifestyle adjustments. This book is an inspiring blueprint for anyone who wants to lead a long, healthy life.

Izabella Wentz, PharmD, FASCP, #1 *New York Times*
bestselling author of *Hashimoto's Protocol*

Dr. Nandi has impressed me on so many levels. His true passion for health and his ability to inspire those around him makes him such a great role model to so many. In his book, *Ask Dr. Nandi*, he identifies five areas we can focus on to diminish stress and inflammation, add purpose and belonging, and put clean foods into our bodies. By simply paying attention and making a few lifestyle changes, you can add so much to your days—more friends, more fun, stronger communities and a longer healthier life.

Kellyann Petrucci, MS, ND, *New York Times* bestselling author of
Dr. Kellyann's Bone Broth Diet and
Dr. Kellyann's Bone Broth Cookbook

ASK
DR. NANDI

5 Steps to Becoming Your Own #HealthHero
for Longevity, Well-Being, and a Joyful Life

PARTHA NANDI, MD, FACP

NORTH
STAR
WAY

New York   London   Toronto   Sydney   New Delhi

North Star Way
An Imprint of Simon & Schuster, Inc.
1230 Avenue of the Americas
New York, NY 10020

First North Star Way hardcover edition September 2017

NORTH STAR WAY and colophon are trademarks of Simon & Schuster, Inc.

For information about special discounts for bulk purchases, please contact Simon & Schuster Special Sales at 1-866-506-1949 or business@simonandschuster.com.

The North Star Way Speakers Bureau can bring authors to your live event. For more information or to book an event, contact the North Star Way Speakers Bureau at 1-212-698-8888 or visit our website at www.thenorthstarway.com.

Interior design by Davina Mock-Maniscalco

Manufactured in the United States of America

10   9   8   7   6   5   4   3   2   1

Library of Congress Cataloging-in-Publication Data
Names: Nandi, Partha, author.
Title: Ask Dr. Nandi : 5 steps to becoming your own healthhero for longevity, well-being, and a joyful life / Partha Nandi, MD, FACP.
Description: First North Star Way hardcover edition. | New York : North Star Way, 2017.
Identifiers: LCCN 2017021658 (print) | LCCN 2017029241 (ebook) |
Subjects: LCSH: Self-care, Health—Popular works. | Health—Popular works. |
Medicine, Preventive—Popular works. | BISAC: HEALTH & FITNESS / Healthy Living. |
   MEDICAL / Alternative Medicine. | SELF-HELP / Personal Growth / General.
Classification: LCC RA776.95 (ebook) | LCC RA776.95 .N36 2017 (print) | DDC 613—dc23
LC record available at https://lccn.loc.gov/2017021658

ISBN 978-1-5011-5681-6
ISBN 978-1-5011-5683-0 (ebook)

CONTENTS

MY FIRST #HEALTHHEROES

Namaste is a beautiful word in the Hindi language.

It means "The light in me honors the light in you."

Namaste is not the first word you expected to hear, I know. It's not the word bandied about by most medical doctors, but it is the first word you'll hear from me. It is also the word I return to over and over in my mind as I treat my patients. It is the *only* word that truly describes the healer's art, a meeting of light between souls that makes them both better and stronger. I have seen this healing take place in my work repeatedly. It is almost impossible to describe and awesome to see. In this moment, our roles become switched.

My patient stands before me, a newly minted #healthhero whose light shines.

That light is a divine sign of your best you. With pills and triage, we've forgotten that if you have your health, you have everything, another old—even ancient—piece of wisdom proved true endlessly. Little is possible without your health. Too many of us walk around limping, literally or figuratively. Something isn't right in our life. You wake up with a stiff neck too many times and have too much time on your hands—or too little. You don't sleep well. You are stressed, suffer internal inflammation, and develop illness. Your relationships suffer. So does your work. Isolation and depression set in. How do you get reconnected to the light?

I've spent countless hours in thought. I have observed, questioned, and pulled survivors of catastrophic illness onstage during lectures in hopes of understanding what held them together through such an ordeal. What was in their character and outlook that allowed them to overcome such a threat? How did they handle such a huge disruption to their life? I have spoken to colleagues, philosophers, and spiritual leaders. Themes began to emerge: hope, courage, a sense of purpose, a positive outlook, dedication to other human beings, and a fighting spirit. Their #tribe gathered around them to provide support and the saying "If you have your health, you have everything" took on new meaning. It was the wellspring from which goodness flowed.

Five areas of life began to show themselves as constants in these great achievers: a sense of purpose; a balanced approach to food and exercise; being part of a #tribe for support, encouragement, engagement, and bonding; and cultivating a sense of spirituality—simply a belief that they are connected to something greater than themselves.

Beyond the machines and chemistry, those five areas were often the difference between a successful outcome and a life overtaken by illness. Those five areas didn't require money, only commitment and heart. I began to look inside my own life and realized I had instinctively made some of these successful moves. Others took years of work. But once you see the simplicity of these ideas and manage to put them into action, the rewards are too valuable to put a price on any of it.

At *Ask Dr. Nandi*, we came to the term #healthhero as a way to describe these glorious survivors, most still thriving. These people had literally saved their own lives (with help, of course) by making their health the number one priority in their lives. Their experience with the lack of health made clear the devastation awaiting those who took it for granted.

The #healthhero puts health first. It's that simple. With an attitude of prevention and a commitment to the well-being of others, the #healthhero builds. This is a way of life that is deeply satisfying and transcends the cacophony of the twenty-first century. The #healthhero doesn't fall for fad diets and wrinkle creams. The #healthhero is occupied with a greater endeavor: making a more positive world.

None of these quiet ideas will make the six o'clock news like the Jarvik artificial heart or the first face transplant, but the impact is just as newsworthy. The right foods now turn off DNA that causes disease. Reducing stress reduces the inflammation that bubbles up into a heart episode or other cardio event. A sense of purpose and the support of like-minded individuals add years to life. Talking, laughing, and playing—making essential connections with other human beings is a must. We are social animals. We were built that way and then disappeared into high-rises and the suburbs. Social media seemed helpful, yet the deep yearning for connection remains. Listening and being listened to are skills the #healthhero should always be developing. Because at the end of everything, perhaps the most important phrase we long to hear is not "I love you" but "I hear you." In the #healthheroes world, no one is unheard and no one is alone. We are here together. This is what I can do for the people in my life. This is how I can honor and help them.

Like so many #healthheroes, I went through my own physical ordeal at a very early age. When I was faced with a deadly illness at age six, two great men—my father and my doctor—swooped in and gave me my first models for #healthheroes. These men stayed by my side and taught me about who I would become.

MY #HEALTHHERO BEGINNING

It was late fall in Bangalore, India. I was a normal six-year-old running wild in this ancient city of 8 million, having a great time with my family and friends. I craved activity and loved school, sports, and music. Then one day I began to have joint pains acute enough to keep me from doing all the activities I loved. No more cricket, running with my friends, or playing with my sister.

I was not improving. My mother insisted on finding a specialist, so my father took me to a man in a big office. I will never forget Dr. Chandrashekhar. He examined me and spoke kindly to me. He then told my father that I had rheumatic fever, a potentially life-threatening disease of the joints and heart. I had to be hospitalized that very day, on Christmas Eve.

I was shocked. I went with my dad to the hospital and stayed for ten days. My mother stayed with me all day while my sister was at school and my father was there every day and night through this difficult time. I was scared and unsure, and my dad was my rock and inspiration. I then understood how important a father is in a child's life. I wanted to be just like him.

Dr. Chandrashekhar saw me daily and his efforts saved my life. He showed compassion, strength, and knowledge, traits important for a six-year-old boy to see. I was on bed rest for a year, with homeschooling. That experience continues to shape me today and, in my imagination, I still see Dr. Chandrashekhar and my parents walking the halls of that hospital, coming toward my room. They were true #healthheroes, flying to my rescue; I can almost see the large red *S* on their chest. My dad was there day in and day out, talking to the doctor, comforting me, and coordinating the schedules of all the #healthheroes who cared for me and inspired me to heal.

My life's course was set: I wanted to be this kind of hero, a #healthhero! These #healthheroes took me on their shoulders and carried me out of that tiny dark world of illness into a state of health and well-being. What a privilege to be this type of hero, to care for folks when they are ill, vulnerable, and afraid. I wanted to be there, a #HealthHero, present for patients when their worlds stopped.

Many years later when my dad became very ill with a crippling stroke, I remembered the sacrifices he made during his life, including never leaving my side while I was in the hospital. When he in turn had a lengthy stay in the hospital seven years ago, I never left his side. With a full-time medical practice and a new fiancée, balancing everything was challenging; but I knew what was the right thing to do. My babuni (father) taught me at a young age the true meaning of family! He would never leave me and I surely would never leave him. No one taught me more about the character and dedication of the #healthhero than my babuni. He lit my way.

Just as had happened with my illness many years ago, my family rallied together and cared for my father. My sister and mom stayed with Babuni during the day, and I stayed with him at night. My sister Mohua sacrificed tremendously to care for him. When he fell ill, she had a thriving soup and sandwich restaurant in a booming downtown area. She ended up selling the business in order to take care of my father full-time. She too is a #healthhero, willing to change everything to keep a loved one recovering and healthy.

THE CIRCLE OPENS

When I ask my young patients about their heroes, they typically speak of a sports star, actor, or singer. Some speak of their parents. Then I pose this question to them:

"What if you were your own hero? What if you made your health the most important part of your life?"

Charles is a patient that I met a decade ago, when he was diagnosed with tonsillar cancer. Since that time, he has successfully been treated for and overcome seven cancers. Charles saw his health and well-being as his top priority. He became an expert about the prevention and treatment of his disease. He didn't give up and he didn't stop learning about how to overcome his enemy, cancer. Charles had become a #healthhero.

And he is not alone. Others have become their own #healthhero and learned the importance of advocacy, education, empowerment, and knowledge. My mission was clear.

We started our television show, *Ask Dr. Nandi,* to tell Charles's story as well as other stories of health and healing. I love my patients and their courage, determination, and sheer will. I am proud and honored to help them in their time of need. I share this sentiment with my life partner, and together we are inspired to improve the lives of others. Just as I do with my patients in my office and in the hospitals where I practice, my goal grew and I wanted to reach a larger audience and impact health on a global level.

I teach my patients and viewers successful methods of advocating for their loved ones and themselves to achieve better health and well-being. To know better is to do better. I began to understand that I wanted to offer people health information so that they might have the know-how to stay healthy. I listened to my family state their intentions—to care and support us in all times, good or bad—and watched them follow through with action. They never let me down and I will never let them down. It is my passion and mission. I've just expanded what I learned in my childhood, the gifts I was given. It gives me great pleasure and purpose to enrich the lives of my neighbors, friends, and patients, both in the United States and worldwide.

To do better, you must know better! We empower our viewers and supporters so their families can have the lives they deserve and want. We offer simple tools to find true meaning in life, dine in moderation, move with purpose, bond with a #tribe, and cultivate spirituality. This helps all of us thrive, living an empowered, enriched life. These are the secrets of those all over the planet—from North America to Asia—who live long, healthy, meaningful lives!

This book is dedicated to helping anyone on the road to a better life; it contains the day-to-day basics to maintain your health and what to do when you are hit by a crisis. This book is dedicated to the unknown #healthheroes everywhere who just need a little direction, some support, and great information to earn their capes. We want to set them free and watch them fly off, healthy and strong, better and smarter.

Throughout this book, I use the word *#healthhero* so often that I'm hoping by the end of the book, #healthhero will be interchangeable with *you*. My hope is that you remember your heroes and take them inside you, adopting their ways and their strength. You then turn and create new heroes through your attitude and effort. Think of it as fighting zombies, creating vibrancy and life wherever you go. You'll need powerful words to match your deeds and fend off illness and disease—scary zombies indeed!

THE NANDI PLAN

This book is designed to open your mind to the newest preventive medicine on the planet. It requires no machines, no sharp tools, nothing to force air in and out of lungs—in short, all the tools of my physician's trade. Strange for a medical doctor to bring such news, but as you read about my beginnings, East/West medicine is a part of my DNA.

I no longer wanted to just "fix" people and then wait for them to come back in for another "fix." I wanted to heal, in the truest sense. And that healing comes from within the human body and soul, mysterious despite all our science and understanding and eons of study. And here we are again, back at the beginning, awash in the mysteries of what drives human longevity.

In the midst of rigorous medical training, I began to look deeply at what drove my own life—those I loved, my work, career, and passions, and my feelings for my community, country, and planet. I read mega-studies that took years of data and simply looked at the findings through a different lens: attitude and longevity; community and health; purpose and mortality rate, disease and isolation—the list goes on.

After sorting through reams of information and shifting theories—medical texts, clinical training, colleagues, seminars, cutting-edge testing and treatment protocols—a light went on, so to speak. I was interviewing a stage full of survivors—those who had cancer or severe diabetes, heart attack victims, severe depressives—and it hit me. All the reading and thinking and questioning boiled down to this stage filled with remarkable souls. They lived because it became their sense of purpose, their reason to be. They stood up and said, "I am my own #healthhero and I want to live my best life." They gathered the expertise and support they needed. And they refused to give up. They fought with their *minds*, a lifesaving medicine available to everyone.

While I, as a physician, could repair a bleeding ulcer, was I really enhancing someone's life for the short term or the long? Had I identified the *cause* or just sent another patient back to run on the hamster wheel of poor nutrition, triage medicine, decreased energy, depressed mood, and a compromised life? Many doctors—fine people who truly want to heal—strive to free themselves and their patients from the matrix of ineffective health care.

The Nandi Plan is one of *preventive medicine*, using what God gave you—your mind—to steer the ship. I don't want you to need my services. Instead, I want you to be healthy and free of disease and to be able to do the things you love.

The plan has five areas of focus, all low-tech and all present within your own body. I want to pass on to you all I know so that you can use preventive medicine in your role as the #healthhero. I want you to stay out of doctors' waiting rooms. I want you playing with your kids and grandkids. I want you to advocate for those less fortunate than you. I want you teaching the next generations how to live and continue to contribute to our beautiful planet.

THE BOOK

Each chapter in this book will offer a deep dive into the ideas of *preventive health* and *anti-aging*. The book includes no surgery, no medications, no unattainable exercise plans. All that is here is you—your good sense and your focus. If you put all five areas of good health into play, your life will no doubt reach new heights of success and joy.

Even implementing two of the five ideas will put you in a better place to live longer and healthier. And let's set perfection aside right now. Accomplish what you can. Do it in small steps. Because, really, this is revolutionary thinking—you are not just running to me, the doctor, every time you get sick.

Each chapter in the book will explore in depth different aspects of the #healthhero, this new powerful being, rich in health and knowledge, ready to pass it on:

1. Finding your sense of purpose

2. The Nandi nutrition plan (no dieting!)

3. Movement (Life is movement!)

4. Finding your #tribe

5. Cultivating the mind of the #healthhero

> People with a low sense of purpose were more likely to have a stroke, heart attack, or coronary artery disease requiring a stent or bypass surgery.
>
> Reference: Cohen and colleagues, *Psychosomatic Medicine: Journal of Biobehavioral Medicine*
>
> ———————
>
> With a higher sense of purpose, people lived significantly longer and had 52 percent less chance of being diagnosed with Alzheimer's.
>
> Reference: 2014 *Lancet* study and the Rush Memory and Aging Project[1]

Your mind sets the tone: A positive mind-set increases your life span. Mind also makes all the executive decisions about your life course. It's time to use it for something other than making money or figuring out taxes. It's time to use your mind to make an amazing you.

Wherever possible, I will try to give you practical ideas to put into play in your own life—anti-inflammatory foods, stress reducers, mind-clearing practices, and simple ways to increase movement in your day-to-day life. I encourage you to experiment and find out what is right for you. There is no right or wrong on the journey to creating a #healthhero. Simply be alert for what works for you. Repeat. Throughout, we'll offer ways to think about how you eat, how you move, and how to stimulate your own spirituality and sense of peace. All of these things have worked for me, my family, my patients, and my audience.

And remember, every time you substitute healthy behaviors for unhealthy ones, you suppress disease-generating factors in your DNA. In 2008, for example, the renowned Dr. Dean Ornish of the University of

California, San Francisco, put thirty men with low-risk prostate cancer on his diet. In thirty days, more than five hundred genes had changed the way they worked. Some genes with tumor-fighting capabilities became more active; some cancer-promoting genes were actually turned off. He continued turning on healthy genes and turning off the less helpful by adding purpose, spirituality, stretching, and yoga.

"I see their eyes glaze over," says Ornish of test groups who hear his orientation speech. But for each level of participation the patient undertook—eating, movement, purpose—their gene expression changed for the better.

You are not your genes. You are not what you inherited. Your lifestyle can change and modify function on the cellular level through *food* and through *mind*.

Science is now behind "the glass is half full" belief, and you should be too. Edward Diener, a University of Illinois psychology professor emeritus, reviewed 160 studies that compared health with state of mind. So profound were the effects of positive thinking, it balanced out the devastating health negatives of obesity! His results, published in the journal *Applied Psychology: Health and Well-Being*, amazed him. For example, 5,000 university students were monitored for forty years, and those with a "glass-half-empty" attitude were the first to die. Even animals kept in stressful environments died more quickly than their counterparts in a more relaxed environment.

Diener concluded that we have had cigarettes, alcohol, obesity, and junk food on lists that shorten life. Constant negativity might soon be added to the list.[2]

Now let's look at the first stop on our five steps of the #healthhero and explore your sense of purpose, the reason you get up each day. This is a huge driver for your *mind* and your desire to stay healthy and happy. Purpose also strengthens the expression of positive disease-fighting elements in your DNA.

Chapter 1 is also an amazing tool to get to know yourself better—how you feel, where you want to go. I had to do the same thing, and the journey was both interesting and surprising. But time and time again, our intuition has told us that having a purpose in life matters. Now we have the science to prove it, as we'll see in the next chapter.

chapter one

FIND YOUR PURPOSE

In an examination, your doctor probably concentrates on your "numbers"—your blood pressure, cholesterol, and weight—and whether or not you drink alcohol and smoke. Just as your doctor might not say namaste as you exit his or her office, he or she will not ask you about your activities, what drives you, how engaged with the world you are, or what you like to do. Questions about your sense of purpose, however, might just be the best guide to the state of your health.

In our lives, we've all seen the phenomenon of purpose—short- and long-term—at work. A grandmother passes away a week after her granddaughter is married. She wanted to see her grandchild walk down the aisle, so a short-term purpose lengthened her life. As his life winds down, a historian writes late into the night, rushing to finish the final book in a trilogy, his life's work. Though we do not understand the how or why of this, purpose drives his life beyond its expected length and he publishes the third book at eighty-nine.

Does a sense of purpose really impact health and longevity that much? Yes, it does. Let's examine the impact of purpose on just one disease, and it is a killer. The Centers for Disease Control and Prevention (CDC) tell us that in this country 1 in 4 of us will die of heart disease, or 610,000 people a year. Throughout the medical world, large studies are in process to attempt to understand how the mechanism of purpose and longevity might affect this huge, horrific number. Could purpose have an impact on heart?

Using a technique called meta-analysis, researchers looked at data from ten studies of 160,00 participants, all sixty-seven years of age and above. In a follow-up seven years later, 14,500 of the participants had died from any number of causes, and 4,000 suffered specifically from cardiovascular disease. Those who had reported a strong sense of purpose at the start of the study were still alive, most still healthy.

The findings were remarkable. In the final report, published in *Psychosomatic Medicine: Journal of Biobehavioral Medicine,* the official journal of the American Psychosomatic Society, Drs. Randy Cohen and Alan Rozanski and their colleagues at Mount Sinai St. Luke's Roosevelt Hospital in New York (one study analyzed was conducted there) stated: "Possessing a high sense of purpose in life is associated with a reduced risk for mortality and cardiovascular events."

Here were thousands of people who through a sense of purpose, the #healthhero's first attribute if you ask Dr. Nandi, extended their lives. They, like most of us, didn't know about the link between purpose and health. Those who lived committed, purpose-filled lives were inspired to do more, jump higher, stretch farther. Because of that belief, they *lived* longer.

After surviving the Nazi death camps, Viktor Frankl wrote in 1946's *Man's Search for Meaning* that his fellow prisoners lost their sense of purpose first, then got sick and died. He proposed they lived longer when they had a greater will to live, that a person might actively cultivate purpose—carefully distinguished from pursuing happiness—as a tenet of physical health. Still, modern doctors are not trained (or reimbursed) to counsel patients on their purpose in life. But this idea, which might seem a bit sappy, could be concretely beneficial.

Frankl wrote about *survival* under the most horrific environments the Western world has ever seen. He also identified the characteristics of those who lived and of those who perished. Thus for at least seventy years we have had evidence of the role of the mind on longevity. Your mind, your desire to live, your hopes for the future, your love for family and others—these are factors that promote and drive life.

The US health-care system spends more than twice as much per patient as almost every other wealthy country, owing in part to a lack of emphasis on and compliance with preventive health services. A pound of prevention, as they say, saves the exorbitant hospitalization and surgical costs of draining an infected laceration. If we emphasized preventive care, imagine the dent we could make in that annual $3.8 trillion health-care cost. At this moment in time, less than 4 percent of all health-care expenditures go toward preventive health.

You don't have to be a trained doctor or accountant to understand those numbers are unsustainable. If we don't all get behind preventive care, our world will be difficult indeed. My hope for you is that this book, a blueprint for the #healthhero, will put you squarely in the "preventive" column, arresting disease before it can take root.

My purpose is to educate—on a global scale—about health. So many people are so busy running around and living their life, it's easy to write off aches and pains or explain away problems with sleep or mood. These symptoms matter. These symptoms are your body speaking to you, and a long, healthy life requires that you listen.

Evelyn listened. A viewer in Europe, she watched our segment on atrial fibrillation and realized that the fluttering in her heart was in fact a potentially life-threatening problem. When she saw her doctor, she was promptly referred to a cardiologist and was told she needed treatment right away. Evelyn reported that she was doing well and the fluttering had stopped. The work of the #healthhero is just like that. Each life it touches in turn creates a new hero. She heard me, a #healthhero, educating and advocating, and in turn jumped up and became her own #healthhero, potentially saving her life.

Viewers like Evelyn make this #healthhero jump up each and every morning. Knowing that we are affecting millions of lives throughout the world is a great blessing. I am excited to get started, to share our message with the planet. Filled with purpose, my family and I feel we are lucky and want to extend this spirit to our viewers, readers, and listeners. Our mission is to help people live extraordinary lives, filled with passion, good health, and longevity. This mission drives me to be better, to make sacrifices, and to understand what is really important.

This is not how I've always lived my life. My family and I needed to search deep within our souls to find the meaning and purpose that now forms the backbone of our lives. Although I was always committed (being a doctor takes rigorous training, long days and nights, and a very understanding wife and #tribe), finding purpose has led me to new heights of dedication and discipline. I continued to practice medicine in my wonderful Detroit, and in my "spare" time, my wife, Kali, and I began building the huge communications network called *Ask Dr. Nandi*.

Keeping always busy is the most widely used rationale for discontent.

So how did this transformation start? Well, it took a lot of soul-searching. My wife and I spent many days and weekends asking ourselves what is meaningful in our lives. What did we want to do for ourselves and our family, our neighborhood, city, nation, and planet? Was having the nicest house, the coolest car, or dream vacations our raison d'être, or did we want more? With my father ill and our very young family, our plates were overflowing! Did we have any more to give? I was a busy physician, father, husband, and son, juggling my different roles with some difficulty.

Like Evelyn, we must first listen to what is going on inside of us, what activities we lean toward, what makes us feel fulfilled, and what leaves us empty. So many live a conventional life full of comforts yet find themselves humming U2's "I Still Haven't Found What I'm Looking For." These folks often feel off track or not fully in their bodies, just making the moves. The inner life is out of sync with their outer life.

Why is this so important? Happiness comes and goes, but a sense of purpose transcends the fleeting joys and disappointments of everyday life. You have a higher road to walk and a way to put the ups and downs of life in perspective.

Psychologist Dr. Douglas LaBier describes a "new resilience" at work in the world. Now more than ever before, human beings everywhere are questioning the hollow areas of their lives. LaBier sees a commonality in all who pursue and achieve a purposeful life: ego, like a cloud that blocks the sun, is set aside in the pursuit of clarity and purpose.

People approach purpose in two possible ways, LaBier continues. Some completely reconfigure their lives for service and others see their traditional life as a means to their purpose, a sort of financial fuel for the more meaningful work they do in their "spare" time.

Seeking and understanding your purpose will perhaps challenge you at first. It requires intense listening to your own feelings as to when you are spiritually full and when you are empty. Unfortunately, a soul doesn't rumble like a hungry stomach or this would all be easier. But there are signs, some mysterious, some head-splitting, that will bring you to your soul's purpose.

The Sufi spiritual leader Hazrat Inayat Khan, who brought his teachings from Europe to the United States in the early 1900s, described the mysterious call from the soul: "He may suddenly think during the night, 'I must go to the north,' and in the morning, he sets out on his journey. He does not know why, he does not know what he has to accomplish there, he only knows that he must go. By going there, he finds something that he has to do and sees that it was the hand of destiny pushing him toward the accomplishment of that purpose which inspired him to go to the north."

Call it what you want—faith or insanity—but the man Sufi Khan told us about all those years ago was pursuing a voice in his soul; he was following his purpose, seeking his north star.

Strangely, my illness as a child became my greatest motivator and strength into adulthood. I knew who I wanted to be—a #healthhero—from a very young age. I wanted to be like my father and Dr. Chandrashekhar. I longed for a life of healing and service. For others, the path to purpose is less clear. Role models are a good place to start.

In high school, I had discovered a great man from my birth country, Mohandas K. "Mahatma" Gandhi. He was a lawyer turned patriot who freed India from British rule through nonviolent resistance. He was a spectacular hero to me. He gave his life to serve his nation, and in the process changed the world. He courageously brought out the best in humanity, using peaceful protest, creating more heroes in his wake, such as Martin Luther King Jr., another titan of change through nonviolent resistance. My report to Mr. Glover's tenth-grade history class about Mahatma Gandhi was filled with admiration; my classmates smiled at my obvious passion for this world hero.

I loved souls that craved service and realized that I wanted to be among them. I agonized about how I would manage a family and a career while filling my own soul with service and purpose. I had a wife, three very young children, a medical practice, and an extended family with health issues. I understood I wasn't Superman, but I had a lot of hero in me.

Given my responsibilities, I understood I had to have my entire family, my #tribe, on board if I was going to undertake more in my life. I'd need their support and help. My area of contribution would be health, but beyond that, I did not have a plan in place. For that, I'd need my family.

As we began our discussions about how we could contribute to our world, every voice was heard, even our two-year-old's. My wife is also a health professional and healer, and she too wanted a higher purpose. Our little #tribe would gather for dinner and the conversations continued until we found our place: We would distribute health information any way we could to anyone who needed or wanted it. Our discussions brought our #tribe closer because together we discussed what drove us, what made us feel good, what we wanted to do more of every day. It was a deep soul dive that finally brought up the pearl we longed for: We would do what we do best, only on a global scale. Through teaching, we would create teachers, more #healthheroes helping others live healthy lives.

All of this was fine and good, a little voice whispered inside us, but we were not Martin Luther King or Gandhi. We were a family of five in suburban Detroit. So our purpose was born around a kitchen table and we started small. Kali became the marketing expert as I began a local television talk show on health. Our kids were both guinea pigs and stars, as we had them taste nutritious food and cook with us. That first show was picked up by another network and then another and now it is global. Through Kali's marketing efforts, we reach millions more with live blog posts and social media.

With our minds charged and our hearts full, we embarked upon our journey, a very personal one. As our health communication organization grew, we knew our purpose was true when our viewers began to shape us, asking questions, sharing their lives, and showing where knowledge gaps lay. Their lives became intertwined with ours in the best possible way: one human empowering another. We had found that guiding star.

As we taught, we learned—the win-win of a purpose-filled life—and as our viewers got healthier, so did we. In the *Atlantic* (November 3, 2014) James Hamblin reported on this happy side effect of purpose when he wrote about Experience Corps, AARP's volunteer educational force of over-fifty-year-olds. Volunteers were sent to tutor kindergartners through third-graders in nineteen cities across America. Through their mentoring, those in the Experience Corps significantly raised the academic scores and morale of their students.[1]

The unexpected news from this program was what it did for the mentors themselves. By giving time, support, enthusiasm, and knowledge to these children, the mentors "experienced significant health improvements, both mental and physical"—though I wouldn't separate these two categories, as everyone is one interconnected being and every system in the body influences another. A brain imbalance is a physical imbalance and an imbalance in another part of the body can and will impact the brain.

Tutors' depression rates fell; they experienced virtually no physical decline and in most cases noted an improvement in health and mobility. Some 84 percent reported an increase in friends and #tribe, a strong marker of longevity in older individuals. (#Tribe = life, remember that!) A whopping 86 percent said their lives had significantly improved through their involvement with Experience Corps.

If we want to be happy, we must first be helpful.

No less than the Johns Hopkins School of Medicine weighed in over their participation in Experience Corps. Their program began with fifty-year-olds and above who only tutored in public schools. Johns Hopkins used another set of fifty-year-olds not enrolled in the program to use as the comparison group in their study. Erwin Tan, associate professor of Medicine at Johns Hopkins University Center on Aging and Health, led the Hopkins study that was later published in the *Journals of Gerontology* (January 2008).[2] Within six to eight months of joining the program, mentors had doubled their physical activity and continued to do so for at least three years after leaving the program. Improvements in memory and executive brain function also rose in the mentors.

Lester Strong, a former CEO of Experience Corps, summed up this new research about meaningful work in the second half of life: "Our members know that they are making a difference in the lives of students who desperately need academic help and encouragement. That keeps them going—and healthy."

And therein lies the magic. A grade school tutor is not just a grade school tutor. He or she is actively serving as a #healthhero to that child and to himself or herself. Purpose creates a beautiful circle of giving and receiving in ways you can't even see or feel yet. Purpose is the key, the magic fairy dust to sprinkle all over life. It gives and gives and gives, if you'll just seek it out and use it.

That's what a sense of purpose does. It excites you, energizes you, and drives you forward. Imagine this impact on your life force and the life force of others.

I can see now how my past informed my future, although I could not have formulated the concept of #healthhero at such a young age. But I was surrounded by heroes, and their lasting imprint would shape the course of my life, whether I was conscious of it or not.

PARTHA'S RX

1. Finding purpose is critical in the life of the #healthhero and can increase longevity and decrease rates of mortality.

2. A strong sense of purpose can lead to a healthy mind and body for the #healthhero. Depression and anxiety rates can decrease with a purposeful life.

3. Determining the #healthhero's purpose in life takes time and patience. Once you have achieved this, your focus and concentration increase exponentially, allowing you to thrive!

4. Leading a purpose-driven #healthhero life can decrease stress, allowing true happiness to dwell in your life!

So do you need a television show to find your purpose? Of course not. Our journey is a unique one, made for our individual situation. The fact is, anyone can find his or her purpose. It takes honesty, some soul-searching, and a bit of courage. You have to find out what makes you fulfilled. You need to be truthful with yourself. It may be professional achievement or success at home, raising your family. It matters not *what* your purpose is, but rather that it is yours and yours alone, that it brings health and empowerment and peace. Once you find it, you will wake up looking forward to make that purpose-filled life a reality.

Motivation, once difficult to find, will be readily available, driving you to your goal. Passion, previously not present, will fill your voice and your heart and soul.

It is not your bank account or credit card that makes your purpose-centric life a reality. Rich, poor, and everyone in between can find their sense of purpose and with it, a calm, centered soul ready to meet its challenges.

An experience in Kolkata, India, haunts me. I had just turned sixteen and was on my summer vacation before entering Ohio State. The temperature in the nineties, it was a hot humid day in the City of Joy. I was sitting on a public bus, and color, heat, dust, and noise, the magnificent meaningful chaos of India, swirled into the bus windows and rolled up and down the aisle. As I sat there, stuck in one of the famous Kolkata traffic jams, I peered out the window. An amazing sight caught my eye. In the center of the boulevard—designed by the British so long ago—was a family. The father of the family was sitting on the roadway median, helping his two children with their homework as the matriarch was cooking their meal. They had wide smiles not often seen in the streets of Manhattan or London, seeming quite satisfied with their purpose-filled life. I smiled broadly, forgetting the traffic, the heat, and my "suffering."

I am the architect of my own health and happiness.

What did the family on that Kolkata street have? Certainly, material possessions were in short supply. But they had something much more powerful: purpose and direction. They were living out in the middle of the street, without the four-bedroom house, luxury car, or latest electronic wonder. How could this be? It was possible because *you—not your surroundings or your possessions—determine the meaning of your life.* Despite their economic troubles, that family had a huge purpose: love, education, resilience, togetherness.

You have to define your success, your indication of happiness, your level of contentment. So anyone can have a purpose-filled life, one that is uniquely yours, irrespective of your circumstances. You don't have to keep up with your neighbors, your friends, or even the media gods and goddesses shown on every screen of our planet. You do you, as the saying goes.

This is all well and good, you say. So I know the purpose in my life, Dr. Nandi. How does this help me? As a physician, I want my patients and community to live healthier lives, and at least ten studies have shown how a purposeful life is beneficial to your heart, mind, and soul. That's why this doctor wants you to think about purpose. Let's look at some relevant studies from medical journals and then work on getting your purpose into play in your day-to-day life.

A recent study reported in *Psychosomatic Medicine* by Dr. Mary Ann Cohen showed in 136,000 patients over ten studies that the risk of death was 20 percent lower with a strong sense of purpose, or ikigai.

Ikigai is a Japanese word meaning a reason for being. With increased purpose, you have increased ikigai. If you have a sense of meaning and purpose, your risk of heart disease also decreases. Although this idea seems intuitive, science is finally catching up to our experiences and emotions.

In a 2014 study of 6,000 patients published in *Psychological Science*, the journal of the Association of Psychological Science, Patrick Hill and Nicholas Turiano[3] concluded that feeling useful and having a sense of purpose helps people live longer. The earlier you find this sense of direction and purpose, the better, but the positive effects of purpose on longevity can be seen at any time of life. Even if you begin having a purpose at eighty, it can have an impact.

A young developmental researcher at Cornell, Anthony Burrow, took the study even further, and in an interesting direction. Previous research by R. D. Putnam, originally introduced in his 2006 Johan Skytte Prize Lecture,[4] found that stress increased when people were exposed to diverse ethnicities. So Burrow enlisted a group of college student volunteers from all walks of life to participate in his study. He put them on Chicago mass transit, and at designated stops, each wrote about their feelings and levels of stress. He brought the students back to campus, where half the group spent ten minutes writing down their goals and the other half wrote about the last movie they saw.

Burrow then launched his students across Chicago on the same mass transit asking for notes at the same stops. Based on who boarded the bus, students who had written about the last movie they saw reported stress. Those who had focused on purpose recorded no feelings at all. Besides being a component of being a #healthhero, could this sense of purpose create less stress and more harmony in the world? It is certainly a key.

Few examples of a #healthhero are greater than my patient with seven cancers. He defies nature, it seems. However, he has a purpose-filled life. His purpose is to defeat the cancers. Sitting down with his thoughts, he decided to vanquish the beast that is cancer. This powerful thinking made all the difference. He committed himself to understanding everything that was going on in his body and everything he needed to do to arrest it. Knowledge led to understanding and then to power. I watched him give countless other cancer patients #healthhero support as well.

As a basketball fan for life, I have watched Craig Sager cover sports for the American networks TNT, TBS, and CNN. With his colorful suits and entertaining words, Craig brought life to the television screen, making him one of my favorite broadcasters. In the past few years, Mr. Sager suffered from leukemia and fought the disease with all his might. He passed away in 2016 and I still hear his words. He was—and remains—a #healthhero.

At the ESPY Awards, an American sports awards show highlighting athletic greatness, Craig was given a special honor. In his riveting acceptance speech, Craig said that in the fight against cancer, your attitude and your mind make all the difference in the world. Craig lived a very purposeful life. He loved his family and his job. He received chemotherapy and then worked a basketball game. With this purpose-driven life, he was able to fight this disease in a manner his doctors found miraculous! His purpose inspired others and new #healthheroes were born.

You don't have to suffer from a life-threatening disease to benefit from a meaningful life. However, reading the scientific information that shows the difference that this purpose can make in your health and longevity is eye-opening. When you seek purpose, you frequently meet spectacular individuals who can help you conquer many obstacles. In addition, study after study reports a huge beneficial impact of purpose on longevity.

People with a strong sense of meaning, Dr. Alan Rozanski states in his 2015 study, possess more vitality, motivation, and resilience. Psychologists at the University of Michigan and the University of Wisconsin found that the higher the purpose score on a scale developed to test sense of purpose, the more likely participants were to have routine health screenings! In another recent study, Dr. Patricia Boyle at Rush University in Chicago stated evidence showing a purposeful life protects the brain against the negative effects of stress. Simply amazing and amazingly simple!

Spending the time to have crucial conversations and doing some soul-searching can lead to startling conclusions and simple solutions to benefit your health and wellness. You can extend this to include your family and friends as well. My wife and children have formulated a core group of ideas to help create our purpose-filled life. This helps my teenage daughter thrive during a very trying time in her life, where she is working on formulating her ideas amid the confusion of the twenty-first century. A family united in purpose and meaning can be a powerful weapon in the fight for excellent physical *and* mental well-being. With substance abuse, bullying, self-image difficulties, Internet abuse, global conflict, and community violence discussed endlessly on every news channel, children and their families have rarely faced a time when they felt more challenged.

My friend Robert lives with his family in a neighborhood in the suburbs of Detroit. A busy physician, he is also strapped for time. He and his wife, also a health professional, are committed to a purposeful life in which the well-being of their family is paramount. They have a partner in this life, one seen less frequently in modern times, but with a rich legacy from the past: a community. They have completely bought into the old African proverb "it takes a village to raise a child."

Kids in this neighborhood play together, the parents vacation together, and they celebrate their successes and support one another in their times of challenge. This community thrives in its quest for good physical and mental health, not because of any fancy new gadgets or fancy houses. It thrives with collective purpose and meaning. The families are united in their quest and share a unified goal of strengthening their group. I loved visiting Robert, eager to listen to his stories of block parties, neighborhood cookouts, and resilience in times of challenge and change.

I was impressed by Robert's neighborhood but imagine an entire region of a nation embracing the concept of purpose-centric lives. Okinawa is an amazing example. Okinawans can easily give you the reason why they jump out of bed every day. It's their ikigai, their sense of purpose.

As discussed by Dan Buettner in his groundbreaking work *The Blue Zones,* this is one reason that the residents of this region have such longevity, with many centenarians living there. The ripple effect of the people in an entire region enjoying a meaningful, purpose-driven life is astounding. Okinawans enjoy simple pleasures and don't let hardship stop them in their activities.

In our current world, where change is a constant and many regions lack a sense of community, the quest for a purpose-filled life, one not driven solely by material gains, seems to be desperately needed. What if we can do what the Okinawans do on a daily basis throughout the planet?

It all starts with an individual—that's you—understanding this concept and putting it into action. Purpose informs your life, but it also helps define who you are as a human being and what you will leave behind on this planet—your legacy, so to speak. This legacy doesn't need to be built with dollars; it can be built with the heart.

As I said, seeking purpose can be difficult. Many voices and needs pull you. Hopefully, I can help walk you through a few questions and mental exercises to help. Call your #tribe together for crucial conversations. Explore. The ancient world intuitively understood the power of purpose and science has now proven it to be fact. Embrace purpose as the first step on your transformation into a #healthhero. Learn more about your deepest desires and self while bonding with other like-minded individuals. Listen to dreams. Take your first steps. Nothing is more important to your soul than this.

STEP 1. Find out what fulfills you.

This is the most critical step. This exploration often takes weeks or months, if not years. You must stop and take time to reflect on what makes you tick. Carry a notebook in your handbag or pocket and jot notes as they occur to you. Write reactions to your experiences. All of these things play a part in your journey. Be prepared to ask yourself the tough questions: Are you prepared to change your career, your life as you know it? Do you have a partner who will take this step with you? Bounce ideas off friends and neighbors. Is someone willing to help? If not, are you willing to do it alone, or should you join a larger group?

Once your soul's purpose, your dream, begins to take shape, ask yourself the practical questions: Do I have the resources to accomplish this? If not, what do I need? With each question you ask and answer, you move forward until your plans are complete.

Put It Into Action

Below is a list of crucial questions I used to clarify my goals and purpose. I hope they will assist you in finding the ideas that drive your life.

+ Think back about your childhood. What ideals from then would you like to carry forward into the world as an adult?

+ What from your childhood would you like to fight against? For example, if you experienced abandonment, your purpose may be finding abandoned or orphaned children happy homes or reading and spending time with kids who need special attention or help. Look to the issues closest to your experience and find ways to keep others from suffering what you endured. The good feeling that comes from this is beyond words.

+ What beliefs were you raised with, religious or otherwise?

+ What beliefs do you want to carry forward into the future for others?

+ If your epitaph were to be written today, what would it say? What would you like it to say? What do you think it will say after you have lived motivated by your sense of purpose?

+ What belief do you need to explore for yourself? This could entail rejecting old ideas and exploring new ones. This may also take time. Do not rush it; we are talking about your life's purpose here.

+ What qualities do you admire in a person?

+ What qualities do you admire in yourself?

+ Of these qualities, which can serve you best in implementing your sense of purpose?

+ Who are the essential, most beloved members of your family and your life?

+ What do you think the essential men, women, and children of your life—whether family, friends, neighbors, or a group on the other side of the world—need to thrive? How can you contribute?

+ Look outside the circle of your immediate friends and family and think about your community. Can you and your family contribute toward and participate in strengthening ties in your "village"? Do you need to help create a safer environment? Make more room for children to learn, grow, and play?

+ Are you longing to tackle the largest challenges on the planet? Global warming? Poverty? Water shortages? Fighting disease? After all, TOMS shoes was born when a man named Blake Mycoskie came up with the idea to sell South American, gaucho-inspired, comfortable footwear worldwide and managed to put shoes on millions of needy kids by matching each sale with a free pair of shoes to a poor child. Rick Reilly's "Nothing but Nets" column in *Sports Illustrated* began a $50 million United Nations initiative to buy mosquito netting to combat malaria. A man named Bill Gates took up the cause too.

✦ Make a list of those you admire, people filled with purpose both in your life and without. This list can include famous people or your grocery checker. What they all must share is purpose. If you can, talk to them. Read up on how they built their organization or philanthropy. Use what those who came before you know how to do. Draw upon everything in your life for guidance and inspiration during this phase. No idea is too small, no role model too big.

Your sense of purpose is as subject to changes and shifts as every other element inside you. Adjust your purpose and keep ideas close to revisit and remind you of both what you have accomplished and what further you would like to undertake.

And remember, just as each journey begins with a single step, change is brought by an *individual* who takes that step forward, who moves toward a better future. After all, Mahatma Gandhi, the hero of my childhood essay, simply sat down and refused to work for the British rulers of India. A few others joined him, then a few more. Finally Gandhi's message reached millions and drove the British from India. All this from one man and his simple, peaceful gesture of resistance to an occupying force.

Just as my family and I continue our work spreading information about how to be your own #healthhero, you too should continue reading, exploring, discussing, and sharing your purpose throughout the course of your life.

Once you find your purpose, what makes your life meaningful, then move on to the next step—transforming that purpose into action.

STEP 2. Take action.

Once you've found the source of a meaningful life for you, it's time for action. I would recommend making goals, both short-term and long-term.

Write a list of your long-term goals and tuck it somewhere where you can refer to it often. This is for your eyes only. This is where you work out the meaning of your life and the purpose of your days.

Start with long-term goals, those that require twelve months or longer to achieve. Whether your goal is setting up and running a children's reading hour in your apartment building or working with hospice patients, write it down. This is a place to dream as well. Dreaming is one of the most beautiful aspects of life. World peace can be at the top of your list. You may provide the solution we've been searching for! You can have as many long-term goals as you want. But remember, you are only human; try not to turn this into a bucket list.

Now write your short-term goals in another notebook or at the back of the journal containing your long-term goals. Carry it with you or put it on your bedside table and look at it when you first wake up. Revisit this goal list every day, and ask yourself, "What can I do to achieve this? Am I working toward my purpose? Is there something more I need? Something less?" As you generate ideas and execute them, you'll learn what works for you and what doesn't.

On a weekly basis, make notes on what you have to change to make your goals a reality. In my case, every day I ask myself, "What did I do to add purpose to life?" Whether it was by answering a patient's Facebook message from Africa or an email query from Thailand or counseling a family member in my office, did I help our community and our planet live a healthier, more fulfilled life? This daily analysis will help you to stay focused on the soul satisfaction you desire.

If you become stalled or are interrupted on your path, fall back on the practices that helped get you to this place. Start writing and talking and rethinking the sense of where you are. Your purpose might need an adjustment here or there. It's all a part of the continuum described by Sufi Khan: You may hear another voice in the night, rise, and ride a different way north. Your purpose changes. Don't be afraid of change. If you hear the call, you've heard it for a reason.

Long-term goals should be evaluated weekly. Keep in mind that accomplishing these goals will not happen overnight. Ask yourself, "Am I progressing in making my life truly meaningful, full of purpose?" You may be frustrated by the slowness of your progress, but remember, you can do it only brick by brick, the way everything else is built.

STAYING MOTIVATED TO WORK WITH PURPOSE

Once you have identified and refined your purpose, you need to get moving on it. In a June 17, 2011 *Psychology Today* blog post, Heidi Grant Halvorson, a behavioral scientist in the field of motivation, wrote about the three pitfalls of getting started. She calls this her "science of success," and it makes perfect sense. As you work on your plans on achieving purpose, keep these in mind so you don't get discouraged.

+ You might think, *Write down your goals and success is guaranteed!* Well, not so fast. Remember that brick-by-brick strategy? It must be at work in your purpose. You must have specific, attainable goals and timelines. Granted, they may all change, but the more clearly and pragmatically you work to act on your purpose, the more you will achieve. Without timelines and markers, projects tend to languish and fall away. Again, you're only human.

✦ *Do your best* isn't what you need to hear. In fact, it can sometimes be an invitation to be mediocre. Edwin Locke and Gary Latham, two well-known organizational psychologists, have spent years studying the difference between "do your best" goals and their antithesis: specific and sometimes difficult goals. Evidence from over a thousand studies worldwide showed that when goals were *spelled out exactly* and the *bar was set high*, performance far outdistanced "do your best." Challenging goals tend to increase effort, determination, and focus.

✦ Don't visualize success, *visualize the steps that make it happen*. You have your purpose and the idea of where you would like to go. But you have to see the brick-by-brick way forward to build your dream.

STEP 3. Celebrate your progress.

When we reach another nation or region or enter a new continent, I smile and take in the moment. As I progress in my quest to have a life of meaning and purpose, I pause and reflect on this important step. My wife and I speak about our philosophy of brick by brick. A celebration of our progress helps to invigorate and motivate the soul, heart, mind, and body. I know that I will continue to learn, to make my life of purpose even more fulfilling. I will continue to forge new ways to reach our viewers and listeners. This cycle of celebration followed by the refinement of your goals helps you gain momentum.

At the end, you gain a life filled with passion, in which every day is exciting. Wouldn't that be a fun life? We can do it together, you helping yourself, your family, your community, and your planet to live in good health.

Before we leave our discussion of purpose, the thoughts below are offered to serve as a sort of daily affirmation in your search for what drives you. Dip into them when needed and know that wherever we are and whatever we are doing, we are rooting for you to realize your own vision.

Here are some things to think about as you move forward in putting together your plan to improve your health and the health of everyone and everything around you.

Change Your Thoughts, Change Your Life

Buddha said, "Words have the power to both destroy and heal. When words are both true and kind, they can change our world." Before you change the world, you must start with yourself. Notice the difference between these two points of view: "I got a B on the test" and "I can't believe I didn't get an A. I'm so dumb." If you are relentlessly critical in thinking about yourself and others, nothing is ever enough. The glass is never half full and your negativity pushes away positive people and outcomes.

Every time you catch yourself leaning toward the "glass is half empty" attitude, pivot to the "glass is half full." Even if you don't believe at first, eventually you will. Just keep watching your thoughts, finding positive aspects of situations and people. Soon this will become as automatic as breath. You become a force for hope. You shine.

Stress and Purpose

The exact mechanism for this remains unknown, but it appears that a sense of purpose diminishes stress and adds years to human life. The National Institute on Aging funded a huge study administered by the University of Rochester Medical Center and Canada's Carleton University. Some 6,000 people were asked questions about their sense of purpose. Fourteen years later, those who had reported a strong sense of purpose were still alive and pursuing it. The mortality rate for less engaged individuals was much higher.

Purpose requires commitment and forward movement, but it also diminishes the more annoying aspects of life. Having purpose transcends stress and the horrible effects it has on the body, especially on cardiovascular health and mental well-being.

Overarching Purpose Versus Daily Purpose

Your overarching purpose is the bedrock of your life. It is the primary mover behind all your activity, whether you are consciously aware of it or not. Perhaps you vow to live a life of helping others. Or maybe you want to be the fastest Formula 1 driver in history. Maybe creating and nurturing a family is your special commitment to yourself and the world. Your sense of purpose should inform all that you do in the public or in the private spheres.

That brings us to our daily purpose, tackling that never-ending to-do list called life. Our days are filled with deadlines, driving car pool, working, exercising, and grocery shopping. All these are small tasks that, taken together, make up your life. As you move through your day, accomplish what is before you with your greater purpose in mind. If all your chores aren't finished in one day, move those that aren't onto the next day's to-do list. Stop sweating the small stuff and keep your eyes on the horizon, where your purpose lies.

Also, make the mundane fun! Although grocery shopping can be tedious, I take the kids and turn it into an adventure for all of us. I can be a better father and husband, a better citizen of our planet.

Laws of Attraction

Who would *you* rather sit next to at dinner, a person who complains about the food or one who eats and laughs and tells charming stories? It's simple: Positivity draws more positivity to it. As you change your thoughts and attitudes, like-minded people will begin to fill your world, as if by magic!

Oh, that's just common sense, you might think, but there is something more, something deeper at work. Just as happens in nature, you begin to attract positive charges that help you build an even stronger sense of purpose. Positive thoughts, speech, and deeds are a light in the world, and light draws things to it. And if that light should drive others away, all the better! They probably aren't appropriate members of your #tribe.

Start Small, Aim High

Each journey in life starts with that one single step. If you look ahead, the road before you might seem endless. But once you establish your purpose, the first small action will lead to the next action. Others will join your #tribe and the energy level will rise. You will be able to accomplish more. Focus on the moment, on all you can do today, now, and do it. Write down your accomplishments, no matter how small. You'll be amazed at week's end about the progress you made. The biggest difficulty for those setting out with purpose is the overwhelming nature of the endeavor. There is so much to be done everywhere you turn! Do not blink; do not pause. Move forward. As you draw new members into your #tribe (remember those laws of attraction you read about above?), take on more. Let your purpose build organically. It's not there to cause stress, it's there to enrich your whole being. This is how we've built our worldwide *Ask Dr. Nandi* community!

The Beauty of Failure

After my #tribe and I had worked through our sense of purpose and had begun work in earnest on *Ask Dr. Nandi,* we met many challenges and missed others. Daily, our short-term purpose was interrupted by a missed television cue, a server shutting down, or a sneeze in the middle of taping. We began to speak to sponsors. Some of our pitches were met with wild enthusiasm, others not. We learned and refined our presentations. Later we laughed about our mistakes, but we learned from them. Oh, boy, did we learn. Our mistakes made our #tribe grow smarter, stronger, better at what we do. Failure is the most powerful exercise to build a strong spirit.

False Starts and Refinement

I was lucky I had a serious illness at six years old. Although I had no clue about it at the time, my course was set. It would take many years to put it all together, but *Ask Dr. Nandi,* with its reach into over eighty million homes, was born in my bed in that hospital in India so many years ago. I remember how frightened and alone I felt. I also remember the efforts and sacrifices of my father and doctor. I was little. They were big and strong and seemed to know everything. I wanted that; I wanted to be a #healthhero. What a feeling that must be, I thought. To save! To heal! I didn't have the words yet to describe Dr. Chandrashekhar and my babuni's efforts, but now I know who they were. They were my own #healthheroes sent to teach and heal me.

As I grew, I tried many different things and pursued many passions. I kept thinking back on this experience, and an idea of who and what I wanted to be took shape. I entered medical school with the intention of practicing medicine. I did not enter medical school to create a media organization. But I learned as my #tribe and I refined our sense of purpose—to take sound health information to the world—we needed to communicate to large numbers of people quickly. We refined our definition of #healthhero.

From Adversity Comes Success

Your environment and the images you see day in and day out shape your thoughts, feelings, and of course, sense of purpose. You might feel defeated by pictures of suffering, crime, and war. I usually diagnose this as "an excess of TV news." But turn in a different direction with a different awareness and opportunity shows itself everywhere.

A report on the high rate of illiteracy becomes an opportunity for the #healthhero, an invitation to get involved in one-on-one education. Global warming, the greatest challenge of this generation, feels overwhelming. Yet if you do just a little research, you'll understand the impact of agribusiness on the atmosphere. Just one meatless meal a week will make a difference. From there, our #healthhero might start a neighborhood meatless-night buffet, a composting group, and a car pool to the farmers' market. If more and more Americans give up meat for one meal a week, the effects on reversing global warming would have a large impact.

Create an Avenue of Heroes

From the second our lungs grab at that first gulp of oxygen in the delivery room, we rely on others to teach us. That fact never ever changes. From my patient fighting seven cancers to Gandhi, I am always adding #healthheroes I admire to my list. I read about their lives and look for ideas to put to work myself. I walked the townships of South Africa, deeply moved by the health advocates I met there. I sometimes hear their words as I move through my life so far away in Detroit. A car shot past me on the highway and I was suddenly reminded of the two nuns I had heard about. When Ebola broke out in West Africa, they got money for a secondhand car from an American donor, filled it with liquid bleach, and drove straight into the hot zone. Their reasoning? "Our people are in trouble!" was all they said.

Heroism and nobility are all around you. Whether it's the single mom fighting for a safe place to raise her children or doctors and nurses on the front line battling the deadliest diseases in memory, #healthheroes are there. When you see a story that catches your eye, save it or take note. Think about your role models. Look. Learn from them. Your teachers are ready if you are.

Purpose That Feels Good Is Good

Helping others makes us good. Why? In a 2013 article in *Psychological Science* entitled "How Positive Emotions Build Physical Health," Bethany E. Kok and her colleagues published illuminating research. Why positive emotion affects health so greatly was not understood. Yet they found a kind of upward spiral dynamic created between positive emotions and health, and the spiral was mediated through how people perceived their social bonds.

Lead investigator Barbara Fredrickson, a professor of psychology at the University of North Carolina, recruited sixty-five of the university's faculty and staff to participate in a study about meditation and stress. Half the group was assigned to take an hour-long class in loving-kindness meditation once a week for six weeks. They were instructed to think warm thoughts about themselves and others, such as *may you feel safe, may you feel happy, may you feel healthy, may you live with ease.* The other half of the group was put on a waiting list.

Each group was tested on their heart-rate variability, an indicator of how well the heart matches changes in breathing. The higher the heart-rate variability, the healthier the heart. In control of all this is the vagus nerve. This nerve also seems to have an impact on regulating glucose levels and immune response.

This vagus nerve, of all the crazy things, also connects directly to nerves that tune our ears to speech, coordinate eye contact, and regulate emotional expressions. The vagus also influences the release of oxytocin, a hormone important in social bonding.

For two months, all the participants kept careful notations of the daily amount of prayer and meditation they logged as well as of their feelings of positivity and negativity.

Those who practiced loving-kindness had a more toned vagus nerve and were therefore healthier and happier. Their breathing and heart rates matched rapidly, indicating a healthy cardiovascular system. Their ability to bond strengthened the nerve as well.

So if you want to work your vagus nerve, don't go to the gym. Meet with your #tribe and love them. Throw a dinner party and laugh. Help others. Connect with humankind for a healthier you!

Purpose and Balance

Later, we'll talk about finding the spiritual calm that comes with developing a sense of purpose and the #healthhero inside. Having purpose in and of itself puts life in perspective; you are less likely to be overwhelmed by any one event if you have overarching goals that continue to inspire you no matter what goes on. I remember bumping into my friend Nancy. She was on her way to read at our library, just as she did every Saturday morning. I asked her how she was.

She said, "Oh, fine. I got laid off yesterday, though."

I was dumbfounded! Here was my neighbor, fresh from what was no doubt a difficult or perhaps devastating event, and she was on her way to read to the neighborhood children! I said as much and she answered with a simple "I wouldn't miss my kids!"

She kept her eyes on the prize—helping others—and believed in herself. She got out of bed after a really bad day and followed through on her purpose. Now that's a #healthhero!

Now that you are filled with the inspiration of a meaningful life, you need your body to function optimally. As a #healthhero in training, you have to supply your engine with the right fuel, the good stuff! In chapter 2, we explore the food habits of the #healthhero. Remember, the food that you eat is critical to your health and wellness. It is medicine and life.

The next chapter explores how the inhabitants of the San Blas Islands off the Panama coast very rarely suffer from high blood pressure and heart disease. Their rate of heart disease is only 9 out of 100,000 people, compared to 83 per 100,000 among nearby Panamanians on the mainland! Let's find out how you can get the #healthhero nutrition plan for optimal health and longevity.

chapter two

THE #HEALTHHERO NUTRITION PLAN

First, the good news. Our planet is so rich and diverse in natural foods and nutrients, we can eat an exciting, flavorful, healthy diet that will never bore us. Food has a huge impact on health and serves as a focus for some of our most joyous bonding moments. Food is celebration and food is comfort and love. Healthy foods are also the right fuel for optimal body function, circumventing illness and premature death.

Now the less good news: Most of the planet needs a new diet. Our large fish are chock-full of heavy metals; agribusiness grows food filled with chemicals and pesticides that is low in nutritional value; fish farms feed their stock unnatural cheap ingredients, raising less nutritious and often sickly fish that can jump into the larger ecosystem and harm ocean ecology; and livestock is nursed on growth hormones and their feedlots create more carbon dioxide than all the transportation on earth—18 percent more, actually.

Henning Steinfeld, chief of the United Nations Food and Agriculture Organization, Livestock Information and Policy Branch, and senior author of the report on carbon dioxide gases and modern animal husbandry, says, "Livestock are one of the most significant contributors to today's most serious environmental problems. Urgent action is required to remedy the situation."

With increased prosperity, people are consuming more meat and dairy products every year. Global meat production is projected to more than double from 229 million tons in 1999/2001 to 465 million tons in 2050, while milk output is set to climb from 580 to 1,043 million tons.

Sure, pounds might melt away on Atkins or Paleo, but red meat is a killer when too much protein is loaded in the body. In the March 4, 2014, issue of *Cell Metabolism*, Dr. Valter Longo, professor of gerontology and biological sciences at the University of Southern California, reported findings on protein research in a group of 6,831 individuals aged fifty to sixty-five. More than 20 percent of their diet consisted of protein. Eighteen years later, those who ate large amounts of protein were four times more likely to suffer certain cancers and diabetes.

"We studied simple organisms, mice, and humans and provide convincing evidence that a high-protein diet—particularly if the proteins are derived from animals—is nearly as bad as smoking for your health," said Dr. Longo.

For those over sixty-five, protein had the opposite effect: Their risk of dying from cancer was decreased by 60 percent. Why the huge shift? Perhaps the answer lies, according to researchers, in the growth factor IGF-1. As humans age and begin to shrink, the added protein stimulates IGF-1, increasing longevity.

The investigators predict that a diet with moderate amounts of high-quality protein that is also relatively low in fat and high in complex carbohydrates will yield the best metabolic health and the longest life. *And that means you should get your protein mainly from plants.*

Sure, skinless chicken or fish are magnificent low-fat choices for protein, but it is the vegetables and grains that will provide the most protein, in complex carbohydrates, throughout every meal, day after day. A huge world of choice lies before the #healthhero in tune with healthy eating.

FLAVOR MEANS NUTRITION

Just do the taste test to understand the food sources in this country. Buy the juiciest-looking tomato you can at your commercial grocery store, the plumper the better. Then swing by your neighbor's garden or the farm stand and get another tomato. Do a side-by-side taste test and you'll know everything you need to know.

Our produce contains less nutrition than the foods our parents and grandparents ate just fifty years ago. A landmark University of Texas study in 2004 tracked a fifty-year span and measured the levels of six nutrients—protein, calcium, phosphorus, iron, vitamin B_2, and vitamin C—in a general selection of produce. All had measurable declines, and the losses ranged from 6 to 38 percent. Fifty years ago, you ate one orange. Today you would have to eat eight oranges to receive the same amount of nutrition.

Sadly, companies that provide food to Americans are concerned about shipping and shelf life—the financial bottom lines—and not the nutrition of their product or its impact on your body. Never forget, the longer any produce (and that includes herbs) is out of the ground, traveling or sitting on the shelf the more nutritional value it loses by the minute, the hour, the day.

Modern food is also grown in substandard soils around the world. Farming and pesticides have depleted the nutrients in the soil and added toxins to our foods, contributing to a less vital immune system and an even higher risk from the assault of pesticides. A huge agribusiness operation has one goal—get as many heads of iceberg lettuce or carrots or tomatoes into the markets as quickly as possible. The growing medium, what used to be referred to as "soil," is unknown. Does it even have nutrients? We assume so, but far fewer than we imagine. Making money has outpaced health, a disastrous choice.

Loaded with this information, the #healthhero is confronted with a serious task: how to get the nutrition he or she needs while simultaneously considering the needs of a sick planet.

> *Before you speak, eat, or act, ask yourself this one thing: Will this nourish?*

As an internist and a gastroenterologist, I spend a large part of my day discussing people's diets. As a #healthhero, I place the state of the planet high on my list of concerns. Food choices that fail to nurture and food choices that harm our home (the Earth) must stop. Creating a healthy balanced diet isn't about preparing for swimsuit season; it's about the very future of our children and our world. That's how important your food is.

Many people are personally at war with food: They feel it makes them unattractive and fat. Or they overeat to smother negative feelings, which only makes them weigh more, which in turn creates more guilt. Ruminating about food takes them from the present moment. Life is a battle between the tyranny of superficiality (think bikini bodies and six-pack abs) and the freedom of eating a balanced meal for health and moving energetically through the promises of the day.

As a former president once put it so beautifully, "Come on, man." Why would you starve yourself in a half-starving world? Why would you punish yourself like that? Why wouldn't you choose the way of the #healthhero and say, "I need strength. I need nurturing food. I need energy and health to accomplish my life's purpose: to work, to laugh, to love, to live."

THE PERSONAL TOLL OF DIETING

A patient of mine, Mrs. Roberts, appeared frustrated. "This is the fourth diet plan I've had!"

She told me that on her current diet, she was required to eat protein only. My patient followed the diet but could not sustain it. As with others around our planet dieting away, she experienced failure. And, as we learned above, pummeling her body with red meat was not the best of choices.

Many of us want a quick fix, a way to achieve weight loss easily. This desire has led to a multibillion-dollar business often built upon impossible-to-achieve goals and unhealthy practices. From the Paleo diet to the Atkins diet, we are expected to restrict our food choices in an unrealistic manner. And again, more self-punishing dieting behavior results as restricting food isolates you at mealtimes, creates nutritional deficiencies, and leads to yo-yo dieting and eating disorders that wreak havoc on your metabolism and immune system. And there is more to that list of negatives: Paleo and Atkins both rely on huge amounts of red meat, creating more greenhouse gases and contributing to global warming. We won't even talk about the effect of all that cholesterol on the heart. These diets are just not the #healthhero's way.

A novel study conducted in Finland in 2011 (Pietiläinen et al.) took 2,000 sets of twins between the ages of sixteen and twenty-five and put one on a diet and asked the other to continue to eat in his or her normal way. Not only did the dieting twins actually *gain* weight, but they were two to three times more likely to be overweight in life. Genetics played a far smaller role in weight gain than dieting. Each new diet increases the body's propensity for weight gain. In fact, each time you diet, your inevitable rebound weight gain ratchets up your baseline weight, making you gain and gain throughout life.

That multibillion-dollar dieting business is actually making you more obese, offering you a "cure" while making you gain even more weight! It's a great business model for making money and a devastating model for human health.

We are inundated with television advertisements, Instagram posts, blogs, and Snapchats showing the "ideal" body type, with proposed solutions that are neither sustainable nor healthy. We fall prey to this "drive-through" practice of weight loss and body image.

As a budding #healthhero with a purposeful life, you need a plan that is realistic for your health needs and your nutrition goals. This plan has no beginning or end; it is a part of the fabric of your #healthhero life. It's the way you eat day in and day out. Just as with your quest for a purposeful life, you have to decide what is important for your nutritional goals. Are you chasing an ideal body or do you want to achieve a healthy body at a healthy weight for you? Are your energy levels sufficient to accomplish your goals?

With our family, we have chosen a healthy body at a healthy weight. This again did not come without some difficulty. As a teenager, I often made poor nutritional choices and did not have a great understanding of portion control. Like many professionals, I became lost in my career goals, not caring about good nutritional choices. After spending every fourth night on call at the hospital, I learned to eat what I could find. This often included processed food and not enough fruits and vegetables. I justified my choices by convincing myself I was too tired and hungry and did not have the time or energy to seek out fresh, nutritious food.

As I progressed in my training, my poor habits began to bother me, and as a gastroenterology fellow in Ann Arbor, Michigan, I began changing my eating patterns. I began to understand the importance of my choices. As Dr. Mark Hyman states, "The most important tool in your health is your fork!" With my family, we now make simple choices to help sustain our goals.

No measuring, no counting, no weighing, no food combinations or absolute restrictions are involved in our diet plan. We keep it rather simple. Even with our two-year-old son, we teach him to make good choices. Again, this is not a process that happens overnight but is forged over time. Because we keep it easy to remember—whole foods in moderate portions—it's not difficult for us to be successful in our plan. No one obsesses over calories and food is associated with nurturing and good times.

"Eat what you like, but make sure that you include fruits and veggies with each and every meal" is our mantra. Also, we ask our kids to pick from a rainbow of colors with their choices of fruits and vegetables.

"Go beyond your comfort zone for food," I advise my teenage daughter. Keep food interesting and exciting. Also, pick the spices and foods that help your body not only prevent disease but repair itself.

Food is medicine, and what you place in your body is critical. In a talk about achieving excellent health care in Dubai, UAE, I asked the audience if I gave them a group of pills with no labels, how many of them would take the pills? Not a single hand went up.

Then I asked a different question. "If I gave you a group of foods in bowls with no labels, how many would eat the food?" Several members slowly raised their hands.

The belief that our bodies are somehow indestructible is a bit worrisome. Many around the world feel that their specific food regulatory agencies will take care of their needs. The problem is that these regulatory bodies can police only so much. These agencies want to protect the public from foods that are immediately dangerous for the consumer. They also must weigh the needs of consumers against the needs of those in agribusiness, who want to grow food cheaply and to have it sit on shelves for as long as possible. That formula doesn't usually translate to higher nutritional value.

However, these agencies cannot protect us from our bad habits of eating processed food, which will harm us over time. Obesity, heart disease, and cancers may result when you ingest foods that work against your body's best interests. Knowledge about the foods you are taking in is a powerful tool in preventing disease and maintaining health.

We face the same problems all over the world. Our global neighbors, friends, and family don't know what's in their food. They assume that everything is fine and their bodies will take care of themselves. This is not true! What you put in your body directly affects the performance you get out of your body. One of my favorite sayings is "Crap in, crap out." You cannot expect to get optimal performance if you do not put premium ingredients into your engine, your body.

> *Self-respect is the process of forging habits that cultivate health.*

KNOW WHAT'S IN YOUR FOOD

So the first step in your #healthhero nutrition plan is to know what's in your food. If you are aware of what you are eating, you have real power to make the changes you need. For processed foods, please read the labels. Ingredients are listed in the order of the amount used in the product. Understand the added sugar, the fat content, and the types of fat in the package. Also, look at the portion sizes. A bag of chips may have 150 calories written on the package, but the bag may contain three servings, so if you eat the whole bag of chips, you have taken in 450 calories! Look at the ingredients. Can you pronounce, let alone understand, the chemicals that have been added to the food? Avoid packages with a lot of preservatives, usually long chemical names you cannot pronounce.

Let's look at a typical can of Coke. The first indication that something is amiss is the difficulty you will find in searching out information not controlled by Coke. Bust down that wall and you have this: carbonated water; sucrose or high-fructose corn syrup, depending on country of origin; phosphoric acid; caramel color (E150d); and "natural flavorings." The "natural flavorings" include lots of caffeine.

Carbonated water we all understand, as well as sucrose, or table sugar. But what is high-fructose corn syrup? It is something akin to table sugar, is made out of corn, and according to every health provider in the world, will kill you. High-fructose corn syrup (HFCS) is a huge culprit behind the exploding rates of obesity and diabetes. (Though the exact mechanism has not been clearly identified by researchers, obesity causes inflammation, which in turn causes insulin resistance or type 2 diabetes.) Coke has plenty of HFCS for you. In fact, the company is removing cane sugar from its Mexican brand as a cost-saving device and replacing it with HFCS.

Coke is about 60 percent high-fructose corn syrup, even higher than you might have thought. Drink it regularly and you can easily add ten pounds a year to your weight. And there are mighty forces that want you on that high-fructose corn syrup drip: Dr. Mark Hyman was sent repeated threats from the corn industry as he called out this scourge to human health over and over.

What does phosphoric acid do on top of that? You'd need a chemistry degree to unravel what this does to the human body, but let's just remember it is also used as a rust inhibitor, a food additive, a dental and orthopedic etchant, an electrolyte, a flux, a dispersing agent, an industrial etchant, a fertilizer feedstock, and a component of home cleaning products. While it is not categorized as a strong acid, in its syrupy state, it is 85 percent corrosive and can be used to clean toilets and melt human teeth.

Who would really choose to ruin their teeth after spending that much money at the dentist! Reading food labels is one of the most critical steps to understanding the importance of what you put in your mouth.

On a food label, the first information you need to look at is portion size. It's at the top of the label along with the calories per serving. All food labels are based on a diet of 2,000 calories a day for everyone. The daily value of these calories tells you how much of the key nutrients these foods will contribute to your daily needs. The higher the percentage of good nutrients, the healthier and better you'll feel. Obviously, the appropriate number of calories in a daily diet varies from individual to individual, but 2,000 is a great place to start as you learn about nutrition. If a serving size is ¼ cup and 100 calories with 8 servings in the container, understand that the container holds 800 calories.

Next, look at "percent daily value" on the right side of the label. This is an important step toward understanding what is really in your food. The percentages of ingredients are then listed in the right-hand column at the side. Ingredients such as trans fats, saturated fats, and high levels of sodium are to be avoided at all cost. These ingredients have been proven to have a role in heart disease, high blood pressure, and some cancers.

The other ingredients you should look for are the vitamins in the food you are holding. Is this food nourishing? Make sure it has vitamins A and C, calcium, and potassium as well as dietary fiber. Fiber scours toxins from the body and helps the body absorb vitamins. Fiber also pushes food through the digestive system, a key process for a healthy mind-gut connection. Fiber soaks up liquids, expands, and helps you feel fuller. It's a great tool for weight loss and helps you feel balanced and energized.

The %DV on the label will give you a quick look at whether or not the "food" in your hand has any valuable nutrition. If it is 5 percent or lower, the food has little of that nutrition. If it has 20 percent of that nutrient, it's high. Look for foods high in vitamins and fiber and low in sodium, total fat, saturated fat, and trans fats. If possible, keep these three things to the lowest percentage you can. The %DV helps you balance your intake of foods each day. For example, if you consume a lot of sodium at lunch, try to bring the sodium count way down for dinner. Learn to read food labels in the supermarket and make great choices for you and your family. Not understanding what's in your food can cause a great deal of trouble for you healthwise, as it has for so many of my patients.

Juanita came to my office many years ago. She suffered from intense heartburn, which seemed to be taking over her life. She couldn't sleep and had difficulties at work and home. I assessed Juanita and noted that she was significantly overweight. I also asked her for a diet history and learned that she *loved* cola products.

An endoscopy, in which I place a small fiber-optic tube in the patient's mouth, revealed that she had ulcerations in her esophagus, her food tube. I placed her on medications to heal the damage as well as a dietary plan. In particular I asked her to avoid colas. She was drinking five cans of soda per day.

I told her about the ingredients in her can of soda. She told me she was afraid that she would find drinking less soda difficult. I told Juanita I had faith she could do it and that she should decrease her intake gradually over several weeks. Not convinced, she left my office.

On a return visit, two months later, Juanita told me that she felt like a million bucks; the heartburn was gone and she had lost ten pounds. She had the occasional cola but not the five per day she was drinking when we first met. I was happy that Juanita had really turned the corner and her GERD (gastroesophageal reflux disease, or reflux) had been treated as well! The GERD that had caused her heartburn had dissipated and was no longer causing havoc in her life.

Juanita is not the only one suffering from these drinks, with their baggage of empty calories and acidic corrosiveness. So many students in the United States and abroad get their liquid caloric intake through soda cans and bottles. Schools are serving these nutritional abominations in large amounts. Fast-food restaurants love to supersize or upgrade your drinks, giving you a family-sized cola in one serving. What a bargain! But is it? The difficulty is that our brothers, sisters, and neighbors are drinking all the contents and few understand or ask about the ingredients in their beverages. No wonder obesity is an epidemic throughout the world.

In a Gallup survey, regular soda use seems to be more prevalent in young people between eighteen and twenty-nine years of age. In addition, people in lower income groups seem to drink more soda, people who are the most at risk for obesity, diabetes, heart disease, and stroke. This apparent lack of awareness about the harm in drinking soda with lots of added high-fructose corn syrup is quite alarming. Many count on sugar and caffeine for hits of energy instead of eating real food that releases energy consistently throughout the day. As #healthheroes, we must be aware of what we are placing in our mouths and the effect of those products.

Energy drinks are also replacing smart nutrition choices for many. Instead of eating a healthy meal to start the day, many reach for that miracle can or bottle. I am very concerned about the short-term and long-term implications of these "energy" drinks. Palpitations, dizziness, and chest pain are just some of the side effects that people experience. And always, the crash comes when the sugar wears off. You'll find yourself more confused and grumpier than you were *before* the drink. This is sucrose at work.

One way to combat this is to try to prepare as much of your own food as possible. Knowing what you put in your food enables you to be sure of what you're putting in your body. In the Nandi household, we prepare as many of our snacks and meals as we can. With small children, it's critical to know what's going into their little growing bodies. We also understand that at different phases in our kids' physical development, they require more of certain types of nutrients, whether it's calcium for skeletal health or leafy greens, blueberries, salmon, and dark chocolate to help the skin of teenagers. Growing brains (actually, ALL brains) thrive on avocado, salmon (preferably wild-caught), whole grains (for the promotion of healthy blood flow to organs, and the brain is certainly an organ), beans (for the regulation of glucose—the brain is dependent on glucose for fuel), and pomegranate juice and tea to flush out the toxins that affect brain function.

THE GUT-BRAIN CONNECTION

Stomach flutters before the big presentation, the gut-punch of loss, and certain situations that cause nausea are perfect examples of how the brain influences the gut. In fact, the gastrointestinal tract is highly susceptible to emotion, and that's one of the reasons I was drawn to gastroenterology as a specialty.

The use of probiotics has exploded in recent years. Found in fermented yogurts and drinks and supplements, the bacteria carried in probiotics are part of our microbiome, the thousand or so different species of little creatures in our digestive tract that boost immunity and fight off infection. The prolonged use of antibiotics has decimated many GI tracts of their "good bugs." Today not only do we know about the link between health and bacteria, but scientists now suspect a direct correlation between the levels of good bacteria in the GI tract and autism, depression, and other disorders.

Psychology combines with physiology to create pain and distress in the GI tract. And the sword cuts both ways. The GI tract can send signals of distress to the brain, creating mood disturbances. The distressed brain can send signals of pain to the GI tract, creating inflammation and its frequent companion, illness.

One of my jobs is to identify the source of the problem: gastrointestinal tract or brain. In an overview of thirteen studies reported by Harvard Medical School, patients who tried psychology-based treatments had greater improvement in their GI tracts than those patients who received only conventional medical treatment.

Most often, no matter the origin of the imbalance, GI tract *or* emotional distress, the problem is stress-related. Stress causes inflammation, inflammation damages cells. Left untreated, cells begin to break down in larger and larger numbers and soon, a chronic or life-ending disease has taken hold.

PROBIOTICS

If you haven't been prescribed probiotics by your physician, keep in mind a few things when you shop on your own:

Strain: A probiotic is defined by its genus (*Lactobacillus*), species (rhamnosus), and strain designation, often a line of letters or numbers. Some strains are often used to combat diarrhea. A quick online search of your symptoms should bring you to the most helpful strain.

Dose: Probiotics are measured in colony-forming units, or CFUs. There is no one-size-fits-all dosage, and a lower dose may in fact be more beneficial than a higher one. Begin low and increase the dose slowly. Be hyperaware of your symptoms and feelings. If you have GI tract disruptions or experience mood swings or depression, stop taking the probiotic.

Manufacturer: Be advised that the federal Food and Drug Administration does not regulate probiotics.

One final note on this interesting new frontier of probiotics and the brain: Check the number of *living* cultures on the labeling, keep probiotic foods and supplements refrigerated, and buy new bottles frequently. These are little creatures that live and die like all other creatures. Care for them and they will care for your gut.

If you have a house full of children, the school year presents special demands on nutrition. Not only do kids need to function at their best, the whole family needs a great immune system so every little sneeze and stomach bug isn't brought home to race through the house. Your entire family should add these foods to their diets, not just the kids. The three #healthheroes of the immune system are beta-carotene (the bright colors of fruits and vegetables), which detoxifies cells, vitamin C, and vitamin E.

Some of the best sources of beta-carotene are beets, broccoli, green peppers, kale, carrots, turnip and collard greens, pumpkin, squash, spinach, mangoes, nectarines, sweet potatoes, pink grapefruit, tangerines, tomatoes, and watermelon. Also rich in antioxidants, here's the "B-team" for when you want more diversity: apples, prunes, raisins, plums, red grapes, alfalfa sprouts, onions, and eggplant.

Vitamin C is another immune system #healthhero. You can find large amounts of C in berries, broccoli, brussels sprouts, cantaloupe, grapefruit, honeydew melon, kale, kiwi, mangoes, nectarines, oranges, papayas, snow peas, sweet potatoes, tomatoes, and all colors of peppers.

Another important vitamin for the immune system and health is E. Eat steamed broccoli, avocadoes, chard, mustard and turnip greens, mangoes, nuts, papayas, pumpkin, red peppers, spinach (boiled), and sunflower seeds.

With my teenage daughter, we teach her to partner with us in looking at the foods we are eating to ensure a proper balance of nutrients with fun. We use food to fuel our engines and keep our bodies working optimally.

EMOTIONAL EATING

If we all ate just when we were physically hungry, much of the excess weight of the world would fall away. Food is comfort for many people and masks feelings of sadness, anger, stress, and boredom. Mood dictates intake and wreaks havoc on nutrition and maintaining a healthy weight.

Sure, we all have a bad day every once in a while and console ourselves with Ben & Jerry's. But this needs to be a rare occurrence in our life. Recurrent sensations of being stuffed or gaining weight without noticing are two good indicators something besides food drives your eating.

The #healthhero must cultivate strategies to overcome these feelings and habits by identifying and working around them. If you've just finished a family-sized bag of chips and dip, ask yourself this question: What was I feeling when I ripped that bag open? What happened today that contributed to those feelings? Write it down. Think about it.

The point is that the next time you feel that way, you'll pause before you eat. During that pause, perhaps you will feel the impulse drain away. Perhaps a better way to work out that stress is a walk or some head rolls. Maybe you need to find your calm center after a difficult moment with the boss. Meditate rather than medicate with sugar.

Leslie Becker-Phelps, a psychologist working with eating disorders, suggests her patients wear a rubber band around the wrist. Whenever the impulse to eat without hunger arises, she suggests snapping the band as a reminder it is *just* an impulse and it will pass.

Be kind to yourself. Use food to nurture, not hide.

Cooking doesn't have to be a two-hour affair. Simple, delicious, nourishing meals can be prepared without spending the entire day in the kitchen. The rewards are amazing. Research shows that people who cook their meals are more effective at maintaining a healthy weight and have less cardiovascular disease. Prevent your health problems by using your kitchen, your #tribe, and your taste buds to determine what fuels your body best.

The best meals, according to our kids, are always the ones that we make together. Chicken curry is a particular favorite. Our daughter chops up the onions, under the careful eye of my wife and me. A few tears later, we are ready to proceed. The boys help us in measuring the spices for this Indian dish that is nutritious and delicious, as well as filled with anti-inflammatory spices. I even toast the spices in a dry frying pan to release all their flavor.

We gather all the ingredients and let the kids know what each ingredient does for the food. In addition, we let them know how the turmeric and cumin can help their bodies, including the immune system and overall health. We talk about the vitamins and other nutritional content of the food. We always reinforce the connection between food and health and hopefully teach them about empty calories along the way. (I tell them the story of my patient Juanita and her five sugary Cokes a day. Those Cokes offered no nutrition and plenty of sugar and caffeine, and made her sick by damaging her esophagus.)

At many of my talks, one of my favorite sayings is "Despite my best efforts, I have become my parents." This often gets a big laugh, but it is the truth and I'm grateful.

I remember my mother and father painstakingly explaining to me so many important concepts regarding food and its preparation. My mom's stories were colorful, full of details about the personalities of my grandparents and the time that they lived in; this included the neighbors, the grocers, and the maid. Entertaining, yes. But my parents were doing what their parents had done—teaching their children lessons about how to eat to remain healthy, just as I do now. Establish this #healthhero practice at your table.

By cooking with our children, we are also able to teach them how to work together to create delicious meals as well as to understand nutritional goals. Our family has benefited tremendously from our family cooking sessions. They love broccoli, carrots, quinoa, and peas. They know to eat whole foods prepared simply and beautifully. They understand how the foods affect health. Children should understand how food impacts their bodies and their planet, and the #healthhero is here to help them with that education. When it comes time to sit around the table with their own families, I hope they will continue to educate the Nandi #tribe.

The indirect benefits of cooking with our children are immeasurable. Our teenager cannot stop talking about Twenty One Pilots, her favorite band, and telling funny stories about her experiences at school. My older son, whose vocabulary seemingly increases exponentially every week, tells us about the mechanisms of trains and front loaders.

Our younger son is watching and mimicking his siblings, with intense interest. Almost by accident, we are bonding, forging stronger relationships, and learning to understand one another. Delicious food married with special relationships. There's a magic behind a recipe that binds the dish together—and that magic extends to the family preparing it. Namaste.

Misinformation about food is everywhere. Sara visited my office one Wednesday afternoon, worried if she could continue to work out. She is very involved in fitness and her exercise routines are important to her.

"I'm trying to become a vegetarian, Dr. Nandi," she said with a frustrated look. "I need my protein. How can I get my protein?"

Sara was upset her life would not be the same. On one hand, she wanted to have the benefits of becoming a vegetarian. On the other, she wanted to accomplish her fitness goals.

Without much understanding of nutrition, she did not know that these goals were *not* mutually exclusive. I asked Sara some questions. Did she have any vegetables at home? She said yes. I asked if she liked peas and she said, "Yeah, I actually do!" "A cup of peas contains the same amount of protein as a cup of milk," I told her. I asked her about nuts. Did she like almonds? Yes! She smiled. She was getting the idea. "Nuts have six grams of protein per ounce," I explained.

What about kidney beans? "Do you eat beans, Sara?" I asked. "Sure," she said. "Two cups of kidney beans have almost as much protein as four ounces of beef," I said to my patient. Sara left energized, understanding that she could achieve her goals without compromise.

Sara is certainly not the only one in the dark about alternative protein sources. Globally, many people feel the only way to get protein is through meat. Although meats are one source of protein, they are not the *only* one. Your complete nutritional needs can be met by vegetables and vegetable sources of protein.

The lesson here is to know the nutritional content of your food. Know that broccoli has vitamin C and protein. White beans have 17 grams of protein. Tomatoes are full of phytonutrients to fight cancers and are loaded with vitamins C and A. Carrots, with their amazing color and taste, are packed with antioxidants and vitamin A. Peas will add vitamins A and C and are a great source of protein.

Using the Internet, you can find the nutritional content of every food on the planet. With this information at your fingertips, you can make choices that will give you a great combination of complex carbohydrates, proteins, good fats, and vitamins and minerals. Find a site—some of the best are run by the great universities of America—and take the time to learn about your food. As a #healthhero, share your knowledge with others, hopefully your #tribe at the dinner table.

FOOD CHANGES HOW YOUR DNA EXPRESSES ITSELF

More than two thousand years ago, Hippocrates wrote, "Let food be thy medicine." Again, science has proven another ancient wise man to be correct. Through a new field of study called epigenetics, or how to change genetic expression without actually changing DNA, a newer field called nutrigenomics is exploring how foods turn good genes on and off. That means you are not your past! You can change your habits and begin to reverse the damage at any time. If a gene "expresses" in one direction, it may trigger disease. If it expresses in a healthy direction, you are healthy. Imagine DNA is the gun and lifestyle the trigger. What you put in your mouth switches it on or off, affecting weight, blood pressure, blood cholesterol, cancer growth, and healthy aging. More information becomes available constantly as doctors and researchers press forward with the link between foods and genetic expression.

YOU CAN EAT WHAT YOU LIKE

Diets come and go. Atkins, South Beach, Volumetrics, *Eat Right for Your Type*, a diet book based on blood type, and even the *Flat Belly Diet* all promise great looks and wonderful health. They all give us an "easy plan" of food intake that will help us to overcome our nutritional obstacles. Often these diets include measuring and weighing foods, avoiding food groups, and dedicating oneself to the scheme.

Really? I've dedicated my life to being an internist who chooses noninvasive, human-centered treatment as the first course of attack on digestive issues and weight problems. The diets listed above range from undoable to downright silly. I won't weigh my food or eat only in tiny increments or difficult combinations. The simplicity and nutrition of whole foods is the only "diet" you need. Simply make the commitment to these good foods and eat them in moderation. Don't weigh the food; don't obsess. Food should never be associated with deprivation and a punishing, withholding plan. Life is about healthy abundance and joy.

Barry, one of my patients, had tried almost every diet in the past fifteen years. In this time, he had lost and gained a massive amount of weight, yo-yoing through the period with little success in achieving his preferred body weight and nutritional goals. He was understandably frustrated when he visited me on a cold February morning in my office.

"Dr. Nandi," he said, "what do you think is the one best diet that works for your patients?"

I looked to Barry and said earnestly, "I don't like the word *diet*, sir. I feel it's a synonym for failure." I told Barry that it was possible to maintain a "diet" for a short period of time, but that diets were not sustainable for most people.

"So what can I do, Doc?" Barry asked, a bit confused.

I told him, "Once you determine the content of your food, then give yourself this rule: *Eat what you like*, but avoid supersizing! Eat until you are two-thirds full, choosing whole, nutritious foods. No sugar! No empty calories! Don't waste a one. Food must nurture the body or it's not food. It's something else, thought up usually for profit.

It's really that simple. Nutrition is effective when you love what you eat. That is not to say that you can eat whatever processed food you want at your local fast-food restaurant. Find unprocessed foods that you like and can prepare. Include your favorite fruits and vegetables with *every* meal. You have at least three times a day that you can further your goal of being a #healthhero.

Eat more garlic! It contains hundreds of vitamins and minerals. Besides, no one cares how you smell. It's doctor's orders!

You can't eat a lot of everything on a regular basis. To paraphrase the great food scientist Harold McGee, all the foods would not have been put here if they weren't meant to be eaten. McGee takes us back to the garden, the garden that fills our plate.

A key for success in this plan is to go beyond your comfort zone. When I was a young boy growing up in the southern Indian city of Bangalore, my mother was instrumental in making me a nutritional risk taker. When she wanted me to try bitter melon—well, that was a challenge. My beautiful mama was up to the challenge. With arguments that would stand up in court, she convinced me that the eggplant and bitter melon preparation was going to be delicious.

I started to eat the food slowly but then soon realized how delicious it was: My mother's culinary skills were legendary. Now I talk about the nutritional benefits of bitter melon—it's an immune system booster, provides antioxidants, and aids in control of blood sugar—all of which my mother taught me at age five!

EAT UNTIL YOU ARE TWO-THIRDS FULL: A REAL-LIFE STRATEGY

Supersize me! This seems like an anthem of our generation. From fast-food drive-throughs to restaurants and buffets, it seems the more the better. Our desire to "get our money's worth" has ruined our health and led to an epidemic of obesity, high blood pressure, internal inflammation (the cause of many diseases and an easy way to get your auto-immune system to turn on you). Talk about penny smart and pound foolish: What is temporarily good for your wallet may not be good for your health. Increased cholesterol, obesity, and heart disease follow.

In my #healthhero talks around the world, I talk about the "war" with the buffet table. It seems like we go to battle with this adversary over and over. We are determined to eat *everything* on this table. Is that really "getting your money's worth"? If you eat and eat and never pause long enough to feel your fullness, you will probably always overeat. Why not dine where portions are smaller? Choose whole foods that have been pulled from the earth or that drop from plants and trees. If you love meat, choose low-fat cuts, simply prepared without using a great deal of fat. At the salad bar, reach for chickpeas over bacon bits. Croutons are fine but have little nutrition, so if you want crunch, add some nuts and seeds. Simple substitutions of healthy foods often make all the difference.

If you can, try eating one vegetarian meal a week, even if you have to eat out to get a fine preparation. In India, my home country, we've been practicing the art of vegetarian cooking for many centuries! Up your intake of fruits, vegetables, whole grains, and beans. Those foods add fiber and huge nutrition.

Just as disturbing is the low-fat or no fat movement. Foods with these labels are ubiquitous throughout supermarkets and food stores. Well then, since something is low in fat—or even better, no fat—you can eat double or triple your normal portion, right? Wrong! Most of these foods are packed with added sugar and other unspeakable fillers to compensate for the lack of the taste fat imparts, again increasing your risk of disease.

Gluten-free isn't a weight-loss tool, either, and the confusion over this term is huge. Wheat, barley, rye, and a cross between wheat and rye called triticale all have a protein composite called gluten. If you have certain diseases of the intestines and bowels such as celiac disease, gluten must be removed from the diet. However, these are serious illnesses I see day in and day out in my medical practice. An average person who has never exhibited any of the symptoms of celiac disease (and they are noticeable and highly uncomfortable) should eat wheat and rye. In fact, there is even some evidence that rye bread actually speeds up your metabolism.

The key is that you can be healthy by eating the foods that you love, but the rule of thumb is to eat until you're two-thirds full. Research shows that portion control is the key to weight control while achieving your nutritional goals. Moderation is the key to success. Restricting yourself to certain foods will set you up for failure. In addition, food is meant to be fun and enjoyable, so go ahead and enjoy.

Before we were married, my bride, Kali, had a healthy diet. She loved fruits and vegetables and enjoyed her foods. After we met, I shared with Kali my love for Indian spices. At first Kali was apprehensive, but with time, she and I have learned new dishes that we cooked together. Using turmeric and cumin, we have created some delicious meals. These are also very healthy, adding power to your immune system, helping your heart, and even protecting your brain.

As partners, we helped each other learn how to cook with these wonderful spices. We used them on foods like butternut squash, broccoli, and eggplant. I, on the other hand, expanded my love of salads with new and exciting ways of getting the great benefits of kale, avocado, beets, and even quinoa! Variety is really the spice of life, and this is also true for food. It remains a major character in our love story.

I would recommend picking all the colors of the rainbow in your quest for getting the vegetables you need. If you look at a tray of fast food, the foods are beige and black! Don't be afraid of color. Reach for color! These vegetables give you the vitamins and minerals you need to function efficiently. Brightly colored fruits and vegetables— the brighter the better—have phytochemicals that flush out toxins on a cellular level, preventing disease from cancer to diabetes. Learn to prepare your favorite foods in ways that keep your meals fresh and inviting.

Remember, the journey of the #healthhero is not one of deprivation, but of adventure and passion, even in your diet.

For example, there are many ways to prepare zucchini, brussels sprouts, and bok choy. (Our website askdrnandi.com will give you wonderful ideas as well.) You can choose these vegetables and fruits and not sacrifice. Eat these delicious, nutritious treats until you're two-thirds full and you'll achieve your goals.

As you eat more and more whole foods, you'll begin to find the taste of processed foods strange, almost akin to a petrochemical smell at the gas station. You will begin to be able to tell the taste of chemicals from that of naturally occurring ingredients. The old "foods" will shock your taste buds and leave you hungry again shortly. They are created to activate addiction—sugar, salt, fat—instead of filling you with a sense of wholeness, health, and freedom. You eat an apple and you don't need a mini-rehab to get the toxic sugars out of your system. With a box of Oreos, you do.

Last summer, my patient Bill visited my office. He had a small bag with him on this visit. Bill was not having any symptoms at all and stated that he felt great. Toward the end of my visit with him, he took out his bag of pills. Bill had five bottles, none of them prescription drugs from me or any of his doctors. Instead, they were from his favorite "health-food store." The pills claimed to enhance his workout and boost his metabolism and digestive and immune systems.

"Doc," he said, "I wanna ask you: Is it cool for me to take these pills?"

I looked at the bottles and then answered him. "Bill," I said, "get your nutrients through your favorite foods, not through a pill or supplement."

"What do you mean?" he said, a little irritated.

I told Bill that everything he was looking for could be found at his grocery store, if he would make the effort. Some of the best immune system boosters and digestive aids are in the foods provided by Mother Nature. We have to spend the time to find them. I instructed Bill on how to find out about the nutrition of whole foods. I asked him to make a list of the foods he found in his studies that he loved to eat. From there, we would create a list from which Bill could make food choices. He would get what he wanted from food instead of a supplement.

Far too many of us are succumbing to the multibillion-dollar world of supplements and wonder pills that supposedly will magically take the place of eating good nutritious meals. I'm all in favor of a general multivitamin but am not in favor of the dozens of supplements that some take to maintain their "healthy" state. Often these supplements have additives and elements in super-high dosages, sometimes making them dangerous! As dietary supplements, these are not regulated appropriately. In addition, the body does not absorb these supplements with the speed and ease of nutrients from natural foods. Therefore, they can be both dangerous and less effective than food.

My patient Jerry came to my office with a worried look, concerned that his liver was damaged. Indeed, when he took a blood test, his ALT, a liver enzyme, was quite elevated. Jerry had been taking multiple supplements from a health-food store. The salesperson had confidently told him that it was absolutely safe to take the supplements, so Jerry was surprised at the elevated level of ALT in his blood test. I asked him to stop and his liver enzymes normalized.

Jerry has now diversified his diet, eating most of what he loves and adding some new favorites like blueberries, kale, and cauliflower. Mother Nature's supplements are the best. Use them to help your body achieve the results that you are seeking.

DR. NANDI'S 80-20 RULE

Once you've changed the way you eat, consuming what you like, I want to introduce you to the 80-20 rule. At least three times a day, you have the opportunity to make great choices for your body's nutritional needs. However, eating and food are for your enjoyment and should be treated as such. You should not be paralyzed by having to adhere to the ideal food choices all the time. You should also eat a diverse diet, learning about new foods and ways to prepare them. Food should never be boring. There are just too many choices, and using the Internet, you can find countless recipes for every ingredient.

It's easy to get lost when you have so many options, but with choice comes self-reliance and knowledge, two of the greatest engines of change on the planet. If you can make good choices at least 80 percent of the time, you should meet your goals to be a #healthhero. Using the 80-20 rule gives you room for the vacation to recharge and meet your goals, the birthday dinner for your kids, or the work party. Food is meant to be enjoyed, and if thinking about it and preparing it become a chore, the experience stops being about shared good times, bonding, and joy. *What did I do wrong?* you keep asking yourself. *Nothing* is the answer. Go ahead and enjoy; just be selective about how often you do it.

My father had a life-altering stroke several years ago. He was my hero, so I always found ways to celebrate him. For his birthday, we had chicken Alfredo and lasagna with rich creams and melted cheese. This is how we live our life. We don't have tiramisu every day, but when we do, we enjoy it. We love our food and what it does for our body and mind. Our family follows the 80-20 rule.

PARTHA'S RX

1. Get your head into it. Eating the right way starts and ends with the space between your ears. Once your mind is clear about nutrition, the rest follows. The #healthhero trains the mind to understand the importance of great nutrition and the rest follows accordingly.

2. The way to the heart is through the gut. So true! Many of us whose hearts are hurting try to ease our pain through the gut. Emotional eating is a tremendous problem in our nation and planet. The #healthhero fills the hurting and needy heart with spirituality and purpose, not allowing unhealthy eating habits to artificially fill the void.

3. You are what you eat! So many of us are inundated with media gods telling us what we should look like. Eat to maintain a HEALTHY weight and size, not to match the Instagram and Snapchat images that fill our heads with false ideas of beauty. The #healthhero uses #tribe, movement, and spirituality to understand real beauty and has a diet to match this wholesome beauty, inside and out.

4. An ounce of prevention is worth a pound of cure! So true in the diet of the #healthhero. With heart disease the leading killer of women in the United States, eating until you're two-thirds full and choosing green leafy veggies are critical habits. Avoiding red meat and saturated fat will be instrumental in preventing the clogging of your arteries. The #healthhero fights with her ultimate weapon, her fork, warding off lethal diseases before they can even start.

Not only during celebrations do we maintain our practice. Our young kids often want unhealthy snacks and we do occasionally reward them with treats. Of course we do our best to give them reasons they should be healthy eaters more often, but if they have great nutrition at least 80 percent of the time, we feel we are doing quite well. This flexibility allows our family to thrive. With our sons, we remind them that they are receiving a treat and that treats are not the rule. This reinforcement helps maintain the nutritional habits we want to instill.

In fact, we ourselves often need this reinforcement as well. Instead of feeling guilty about a little "cheating" on your diet, let yourself know that a little treat is okay. When I travel, I often find unique treats that I want to enjoy. They almost always are not healthy and are not a part of my daily nutritional plan.

THE BUILDING BLOCKS OF NUTRITION

So, now that we have understood the general principles of nutrition, what about the building blocks of nutrition? My patients are constantly asking me about three main categories: protein, carbohydrates, and fats. Should I avoid all sugar? Should I have a high-protein diet? What are good fats? Let's delve into these questions and find out what our #healthhero approach should be.

My patient Donovan is very interested in fitness, and he's in the gym several times a week. One visit, he asked me, "Doc, you keep advising me on avoiding red meat. I'm a man and need my meat for protein. I can't do that without my meat."

Donovan is in the majority, if the lines for hamburgers and the abundance of steak houses are any indication. Americans love meat. Many feel that they can get their protein only from animal sources—more specifically, from red meat. They are afraid that if they don't eat meat, "weakness" will result and they won't be able to achieve their goals. Also, many feel the more protein, the better. Donovan also feels this way. Between his protein shakes and meat, he rejoices that he is treating his body right and giving it the tools it needs to give him the muscular body he is working toward in the gym.

I told Donovan that only 30 to 35 percent of his calories should come from protein. Clearly, protein is an important building block of the body. However, lean proteins are critical. Also, fish and chicken can be used instead of red meat. I tell Donovan and other patients about another amazing source of protein: vegetables and beans. The point is, with a little research, Donovan can eat heart-healthy foods such as beans and grains and meet his muscle-building goals while being a #healthhero!

"Doc, I can't have any sugar," says Valerie, my patient who enjoys reading about health trends. Valerie read that *all* sugar is bad! She wants a diet that avoids all sugar.

"So, what sugars do you want to avoid?" I ask.

As with others who ask similar questions, Valerie does not understand the relationship between sugars and carbohydrates. Simple sugars, simple carbohydrates, are not great for the #healthhero. Examples of simple sugars include white rice and candy bars. This is in contrast to complex carbohydrates, such as vegetables and fruits. While simple carbohydrates don't have added nutritional value and just contribute calories, complex carbohydrates are surrounded by vitamins, minerals, antioxidants, and fiber.

Also, many of the simple sugars have a high glycemic index, facilitating the rapid rise in the body's blood sugar and insulin secretion. Your blood sugar rises and crashes, sending you spiraling to earth. Complex carbohydrates often have a lower glycemic index, enabling a gradual increase in the blood sugar levels and a subsequent gradual increase in insulin level. There is no crash, only sustained energy. So Valerie's statements, along with those of countless others who feel that all carbs are bad, have to be qualified.

In fact, we all need carbohydrates in our diet. The #healthhero cape will fly high when 40 to 45 percent of our diet is composed of complex carbohydrates. Again, our hero should avoid the simple sugars and concentrate on fruits and veggies as primary source of nutritious carbohydrates. A beautiful rainbow of vegetables and fruits must be present at every meal, and I would recommend a wide variety of these colorful foods.

Food is love, my wife says to our family, and it's so true as we bite into a delicious mango or slice of avocado. Very few feelings top those you get when you are feeding people you love nutritious delicious food. This comes as second nature to the #healthhero. Complex carbohydrates are a great source of energy and nutrients, and we all need to learn to love them. Instead of listening to generalizations promoted by the media and our friends and advisers, let's look at what science has to offer. Only then will we have true health and wellness.

When I shop in the grocery aisles, I am continually amazed by the multitude of products labeled *fat-free* or *low-fat*. Another popular idea is the notion that *all* fat is our enemy. Supposedly we should not have any fat at all, and many are frustrated and confused at the varying opinions regarding fat. Many of my patients are falling prey to diet plans and advertisements maintaining that any fat will lead to the failure of their health goals.

The truth is, fat is a building block for all of our #healthheroes. We need fat in our diet, with approximately 25 to 30 percent of our food intake being from fat sources. (Our brains are made of 60 percent fat, which in turn creates all the cell membranes in our bodies. Talk about a job!) However, all fat is not the same. We must strive to eat good fats.

My daughter cites guacamole as a great example of a good fat (avocados), as is the salmon curry that my wife and I make (fish oil). Good fat is delicious and helps you stay healthy while building a stronger brain and nervous system.

Bad fat can do the opposite. Saturated fat can wreak havoc on your system. That juicy steak or the lamb chops you crave have loads of saturated fat. Saturated fats, trans fats, and cholesterol build up inside your body. That doesn't mean you can never have a steak. Rather, make the steak the exception, not the rule. Utilize that 80-20 ratio. Have the good fat in nuts, avocados, and fish and avoid the bad fats in bacon.

To help the #healthhero understand what is at stake in the strange world of fats, let's look at trans fats. Invented in the 1950s, partially hydrogenated and fully hydrogenated, or trans, fats kept processed foods such as crackers and cookies crisper and on the shelf longer. It was great for the bottom line of food manufacturers and grocers but unfortunately contributed to the ill health and subsequent deaths of perhaps millions of Americans. Over time—we're talking forty to forty-five years—scientists began to see a correlation between consumption of this fat and a rise in cases of cardiovascular illness, diabetes, infertility, obesity, major depressive disorders (remember, your brain is mostly made of fat!), and cancers.

Finally, in November 2013, the Food and Drug Administration (FDA) reclassified trans fats as a food additive and announced that in the next three years, food had to be free of these fats, unless approved by the FDA. Prior to this announcement in 2010, Americans were consuming 5.8 grams of trans fat a day.

The added sugars in the low-fat and fat-free foods will also lead to big problems for the #healthhero. The amount of simple sugar that's placed in these supposed "healthier" foods can damage your health, increase your weight, lead to obesity, and worsen your cardiovascular status. Again, knowledge is the key. You can't do better if you don't know better! Understand that the general statements on food packaging don't always reflect the truth about nutrition.

DR. NANDI'S TOP PICKS

This list is full of my personal favorites for health and flavor. I'll give you information that helps you understand why they are my go-to vegetables. As you begin to practice the 80-20 rule, eat foods from this list *most* of the time. Explore and research new and exotic foods coming into the market for exciting flavors. Imagine, you can have a perfect mango from Central America at one meal and then pop over to China for a bok choy stir-fry. Globalization was invented in the grocery store! What a wonderful way to discover other cultures and ideas.

So many people don't believe that a plant-based diet provides all the protein they need, even if they are athletes. The vegetables below are highest in protein.

VEGETABLES

Broccoli is full of dietary fiber. Just 1 cup of raw broccoli provides 135 percent of your daily vitamin C. Broccoli is full of phytonutrients that flush toxins out of human cells.

Peas have a quarter of your vitamin A and C needs for the day and are a powerhouse of fiber and protein. You also get a good dose of copper, folate, niacin, magnesium, riboflavin, calcium, and iron. Learn to love the mighty pea.

Kale is the butt of many jokes but has a one-two punch of 134 percent of your daily vitamin C needs and 206 percent of your vitamin A needs.

Corn: If you are looking for fiber and protein, this is your vegetable. It has almost half your daily fiber needs, 12 grams of protein, and a quarter of your daily iron. Higher on the glycemic index, corn enters the bloodstream more quickly than other vegetables.

Edamame (fresh soybeans) are delicious beans with high levels of protein and fiber.

Brussels sprouts have almost no calories, a glycemic load of 1 (that's good; it's as low as it goes), and a quarter of your daily requirement of vitamin C.

Spinach and other cooked leafy greens: Spinach has over 350 percent of the vitamin A experts suggest you consume each day. It also provides a quarter of the vitamin A, vitamin C, and calcium requirements. Chard has double the vitamin A you need and half the vitamin C. Mustard greens, like chard, have double the A and almost two-thirds of the vitamin C. Beet greens have the same: double the vitamin A and almost half the C you require.

Carrots are the king (queen?) of vitamin A, having more than 400 percent of the daily requirement and the color!

Peppers have double the vitamin C needed for an adult to make it through the day. They are also brightly colored, and that means they are full of the phytonutrients that clean toxins from your cells.

Countless other delicious vegetables didn't make the list but are nevertheless essential for their vitamins and minerals—phosphorus, selenium, niacin, manganese, potassium, zinc, magnesium, copper, thiamine, among others—as well as vitamins B_6, B_{12}, E, and K.

Draw heavily from the vegetables above and add squash, mushrooms, bok choy, cabbage, pumpkin, asparagus, cauliflower, lettuces, celery, radishes, green onions, green beans, okra, and as many other vegetables as you encounter. Mix it up; keep it interesting.

FRUIT

All the foods below share fiber and phytonutrients essential for detoxing the body on both a macro and micro scale. All the information below is based on raw fruit.

+ Apples are said to keep people like me away. The reason? The fiber and the vitamin C. Apples move through the system, cleaning it out, and are very low on the glycemic index, releasing their energy slowly.

+ Blackberries have almost half your day's need of both fiber and vitamin C as well as folate, magnesium, potassium, and copper.

- Blueberries, a great source of vitamin C, are one of the world's superfoods because of the power of that color and what it does to cells. Eat these often.

- Grapes should be chosen for their color—the darker the better for those phytonutrients and resveratrol (along with blueberries and raspberries), a phenol that some have linked—though no scientific proof exists—to longevity.

- Mangoes are sweet and colorful (by now I'm hoping you know that color is good, right?). They are also full of vitamins A and C as well as B_6 and dietary fiber.

- Oranges and nectarines are the godsends of winter, and one should meet your daily requirement of vitamin C, color, and fiber detox.

- Papayas are powerhouses of vitamin A and C and are full of color and fiber.

- Pineapple is a titan of vitamin C and fiber. Aloha.

- Raspberries belong to the group with resveratrol that may or not have anti-aging properties. While science investigates, that color is all we need to know.

- Strawberries offer a blast of vitamin C that will satisfy the day's requirement, and the strawberry's color makes it a phytonutrient that happens to be full of manganese. Pesticides tend to cling to strawberries, so wash with even more care than other fruits or buy organic.

Don't forget peaches and pears, cantaloupes and watermelon. Bananas are healthy, though high in calories; I eat a banana on strenuous days or after workouts to replenish the potassium levels in my muscles. Our little ones, however, burn the calories in minutes! Given this fruit comes with its own packaging, it's perfectly mobile for busy kids.

MIGHTY GRAINS

Amaranth has been used around the world for centuries to boost nutrition in everything from soups and stews to candy. Technically a genus of herbs, amaranth has 30 percent more protein than wheat flour, rice, and oats. Vitamins A, B$_6$, and K, folate, manganese, magnesium, iron, and potassium are all here, which makes this a muscle recovery food on the level of bananas.

Bulgur is a whole grain that should not be eaten on a gluten-free diet, and is packed with fiber and protein.

Quinoa has your protein, fiber, iron, calcium, copper, magnesium, manganese, phosphorus, potassium, selenium, and zinc. If that's not enough for you, it is high in tryptophan, the feel-good nutrient found in foods such as turkey.

Whole grain and multigrain breads are the only kinds of bread you should bring into the house with regularity. High in fiber, protein, selenium, and manganese, this bread empowers whatever it touches.

Oatmeal's fantastic reputation is all true: high in fiber and weighing in with a whopping 11 grams of protein per cup, there are few better foods to fuel the #healthhero. Add the fruits discussed above to your heart's content.

Whole grain pasta should take the place of white pasta, which enters the bloodstream and converts to sugar too quickly, followed by that crash. With whole grain pastas, you will get the sustained release of energy of complex carbohydrates. A cup has 7 grams of protein as well as fiber, manganese, and selenium—important nutrients all.

Brown rice falls into the pasta category: Don't eat the white kind. It enters your bloodstream and converts to sugar too quickly, leading to weight gain and that crash that comes from simple carbs. Eat brown rice with its 5 grams of protein and 4 grams of fiber per cup.

BEAN PROTEIN POWER

Navy beans have 15 grams of protein, 19 grams of dietary fiber, and 25 percent of your daily iron needs. Learn to love them and your body will love you.

Black beans have almost the same nutritional profile as navy beans with a little less fiber.

Pinto beans have a huge protein load of 15 grams and fiber to match. You'll also get a quarter of your daily iron as well as manganese and phosphorus.

Garbanzo beans, also known as chickpeas, have 50 percent of your daily fiber needs, 25 percent of your iron requirement, and 15 grams of protein.

Lentils have 18 grams of protein, close to half of your daily iron requirement, phosphorus, copper, folate, and manganese. These little guys are huge in dietary fiber as well.

The above is only a partial list of the world's offerings when it comes to beans. The overall nutritional profile between types does not vary that much, so eat all the different varieties to your heart's content.

Prepared well, their creamy, toothy goodness absorbs all the flavors around them and creates spectacular dishes from Indian dal to Boston baked beans.

MORE PHENOMENAL PROTEINS

Fish holds more protein than any of the foods discussed above. From salmon to swordfish, perch to Arctic char, fish has an average serving of 20-plus grams of protein per serving. In addition, the good fats in fish are said to provide important nutrition to the brain. However, you must be careful as to the source of the fish. A steady diet of large predatory fish will cause the heavy metals in the fish (from ocean pollution) to build up in your body. Therefore, this is more a once-a-week than an everyday meal, and that includes tuna fish and freshwater fish as well. Always choose wild over farmed fish, if possible, but understand that wild-caught will be higher in price.

Lean chicken has almost 50 percent of your daily protein requirement as well as phosphorus, selenium, and niacin. There's a reason chicken breasts are the most popular meat in the United States.

Plain yogurt has 9 grams of protein and a third of your daily calcium needs.

Eggs have 17 grams of protein as well as good amounts of vitamins A and B, iron, and selenium. It is true that eggs are high in saturated fat, a problem for cardiovascular issues.

Cottage cheese will give you a quarter of the calcium you need each day as well as a whopping 27 grams of protein. There is a large amount of sodium in each serving, so be advised.

FANTASTIC FATS

Good fats are monounsaturated and polyunsaturated fats. These fats are shown to improve cholesterol levels, reduce the risk of diabetes, promote healthy nerve function, help the body absorb nutrients, promote cell development, and maintain a strong immune system. The American Heart Association suggests 15 to 25 percent of your daily calories should come from fat—good fat.

Here's the list:

Avocado oil

Olive oil

Sesame oil

Salmon oil

Almond oil

Canola and other vegetable oils

NUTS AND SEEDS

Nuts and seeds are perfect snacks and great for your heart because they lower bad cholesterol levels. Nuts also have plant-based omega fatty acids, fiber, and vitamin E. Try to eat them raw or dry roasted; you can't control the oil in which they were "roasted" if that is what you choose.

Almonds

Pecans

Pistachios

Hazelnuts

Cashews

Macadamias

Brazil nuts

Walnuts

Peanuts

Seeds such as sunflower are delicious snacks. They are full of vitamin A, which most Americans are deficient in. Eat shelled and dry roasted. Antioxidant effects of this tiny food are amazing. Chia seeds, not to be confused with pets, were a staple of Incan and Aztec culture and, unlike flaxseeds, can be eaten whole. A wee superfood that has recently become popular, chia is full of omega-3 fatty acids, antioxidants, and calcium.

Flaxseeds must be ground to release their effects of omega-3 and omega-6 fatty acids and fiber. Buy a coffee grinder or clean an old one: It's the perfect way to grind the flax. The more recently the seeds have been ground, the greater the amount of nutrients.

———————

So, now that you're armed with some ideas of foods and what they contain, including our basic building blocks, it's time to make some #healthhero meal plans. Let's start with breakfast. My mother taught me the importance of a healthy breakfast in my performance at school. Turns out, she was right.

Here's just a sample of how we put this whole approach to eating together. Use it as the loosest of guides and find what works best for your tastes and time constraints. The more you like your healthy diet, the more you will continue to follow it, 80 percent of the time!

BREAKFAST PLAN

Complex carbohydrates: Whole grain cereal.

Fruit: Pick your favorite. I love blueberries, mangoes, apples. You can make fruit smoothies as well (we'll share a great avocado smoothie recipe on page 88).

Protein: Salmon would be a good choice, as would lean turkey slices. The milk in your smoothie also would be good source of protein.

Fat: You can include fat in your smoothie by adding an avocado or nuts. You can also eat either without a smoothie.

LUNCH PLAN

Complex carbohydrates: Steamed or grilled veggies are a staple at our house. Try them here. Our family favorites include broccoli, cauliflower, and brussels sprouts, but include your favorite. A nice salad with loads of veggies and fruits makes for a fantastic lunch entrée. Don't be afraid to put strawberries, raspberries, mandarin orange slices, blackberries, and fresh peach slices onto the greens.

Protein: Grilled or curried chicken or fish are excellent lunch fare. Our family likes cod. A turkey sandwich would be perfect as well. A nutritious salad with quinoa or some other grain would be a fantastic choice or a warm butternut squash quinoa salad, one of my favorites. It is an appropriate entrée (the recipe is on page 89).

Fat: Grilled fish again would fit. A smoothie with avocado or nuts is a cool choice on a summer day.

DINNER PLAN

Complex carbohydrates: Start with a salad. Our warm quinoa salad is a family favorite, especially for my wife, and the recipe is included for your pleasure. This salad is an antioxidant #healthhero. Another good choice is steamed or sautéed vegetables.

Protein: Grilled chicken or my daughter's favorite, chicken curry. Two easy and delicious chicken curry recipes are included in this chapter. Another possibility is grilled or baked fish, such as cod or salmon, on a bed of wild rice or quinoa.

Fat: The good fat in fish would meet your good fat requirement. Also, having nuts and avocado in your salad is a delicious way to add it to the meal and thus your body.

NUTRITION BLASTS

Here are a few simple ways my wife and I have found to add more nutrition to go-to foods in our go-go life:

1. Add ¼ cup of peanut, cashew, or almond butter to any fruit-based smoothie. You increase the smoothie's protein content and provide more fuel to the body longer, creating stamina.

2. Think of granola and oatmeal as fruit and nut delivery systems. Add berries, slivered almonds, walnut pieces, chia seeds, and ground flax to increase flavor and nutritional power. Use almond milk instead of dairy.

3. Detox with a cup of strong black tea mixed with the juice of one

lemon. You'll get a blast of vitamin C while having your cells flushed of toxins.

4. Take a simply grilled chicken breast or firm white fish fillet and sauce it with nutrition.

   In a small pan, combine the juice of 2 oranges and ¼ cup of chicken stock. Bring to a boil, reduce the heat, and simmer until the liquid is cut in half or more. Pour over the entrée.

5. Rinse a can of black or pinto beans and add to rice any time you serve it. The beans add texture but won't interrupt the flavor. They also combine with rice to create a powerful protein addition to any dish.

6. Home-baked goods such as muffins and quick breads should also get several tablespoons of ground flaxseeds to up the nutrition and add omega-3 fatty acids, so prized by your brain and cardiovascular system. The flax has to be ground to release its amazing properties; an old coffee grinder is best for this. Throw chia seeds and ground flax into your smoothies, granola, and oatmeal as well.

7. Add up to ¼ cup of turmeric to smoothies to fight the internal inflammation that is so devastating to cells and organs. Turmeric will color the drink, but the taste is negligible.

8. Throw a handful of fresh herbs into salads or atop roasted meats, toss them with vegetables, or mix them with olive oil to drizzle on tomatoes. Oregano (Greek, Mexican, and Italian varieties) carries a huge antioxidant punch, followed by the next most potent: dill, thyme, rosemary, and peppermint. Use fresh chopped herbs with great abundance—¼ or ½ cup at a time. Brew peppermint tea. View and use herbs as a food, full of nutrition and flavor.

9. Serve ¼ of an avocado, sliced, as a side for every meal. Avocados are a superfood; it's as simple as that. Don't worry about the calories. Your body (all your organs including your brain) will soak that nutrition up like a sponge.

10. As often as possible, prepare and eat with your #tribe. The combination of good nutrition and bonding (don't forget your vagus nerve!) is a win-win for the entire body.

Armed with the knowledge of the #healthhero nutrition plan to fuel a purpose-centric life, you are now ready to pursue another #healthhero goal—to move with purpose. Endless fitness crazes come and go. So what is a healthy way to improve your health and move with purpose? How can you sustain this? The next chapter will give you some ideas.

Below, we share the Nandi household's favorite go-to recipes in hopes they will become yours. We use some of the foods we discussed in this chapter and still more that come and go on our family table. I know it's a bit unusual for the doctor to begin cooking in the middle of the examination, but remember, most doctors don't say namaste either. And I also did it for an even better reason. I hope these recipes draw you back to this chapter repeatedly. Food is that important: It changes your DNA. I hope this chapter reminds you of forgotten ideas and continues to inspire.

PUTTING IT INTO ACTION:
THE RECIPES

Dr. Nandi's Avocado Smoothie

Quick, mobile, and full of good fats, this is one great way to start the day. I make these with the kids and boom! We're out the door.

1 SERVING

1 cup ice
1 cup milk
1 whole avocado, pitted and peeled

Juice of 1 lime
Handful of almonds

Place the ice, milk, avocado, and lime juice in a blender and blend until combined. Sprinkle with almonds.

Dr. Nandi's Warm Quinoa Salad

4 SERVINGS

1 eggplant, cut into 2-inch pieces

2 red onions, cut into thin wedges

1 large zucchini, cut into 2-inch
   pieces

1 teaspoon olive oil, plus olive oil
   from a spray (store-bought or
   homemade)

Freshly ground black pepper

1 cup small cherry tomatoes

1 garlic clove, crushed

1 teaspoon ground cumin

1 cup quinoa

2 cups vegetable broth

1 (15-ounce) can no-salt-added
   chickpeas, rinsed and drained

½ cup torn fresh basil leaves, plus
   more for garnish

½ cup crumbled feta cheese

2 teaspoons extra-virgin olive oil

Salt

1. Preheat the oven to 375°F. Line a large rimmed baking sheet with parchment paper. Place the eggplant, onions, and zucchini on the baking sheet. Spray with oil and season with pepper. Roast for 10 minutes. Add the tomatoes to the baking sheet and roast for 10 minutes more, or until the vegetables are golden and tender.

2. Meanwhile, heat the 1 teaspoon olive oil in a medium saucepan over medium heat. Stir in the garlic and cumin and cook for 30 seconds, or until aromatic. Add the quinoa and broth. Bring to a boil. Reduce the heat to low. Cover and simmer for 12 minutes, or until the quinoa is tender and the broth has been absorbed. Set aside to cool slightly.

3. Place the quinoa, vegetables, chickpeas, basil, and feta in a large bowl. Drizzle with the extra-virgin olive oil. Toss gently to combine. Season with salt and pepper and garnish with basil leaves.

The Nandis' Favorite Chicken Curry

Get some of those anti-inflammatory, life-extending, healthy Eastern spices into your diet. These ingredients have been used for centuries as medicine and in recent years have been studied and proven to decrease the body's inflammation, creating health and extending life. If inflammation is the beginning of all disease, losing weight and easing the burn of too much food and too many unhealthy, bad-fat–filled, unnatural ingredients is a must. Make it a top priority.

4 SERVINGS

1 tablespoon olive oil
1 tablespoon unsalted butter
3 garlic cloves, crushed
1 medium onion, finely chopped
2 tablespoons garam masala
1 teaspoon ground coriander

½ teaspoon dried mint
1½ pounds boneless, skinless
   chicken breast, diced
1 cup water
Chopped fresh cilantro, for garnish
   (optional)

1. Heat the oil and butter in a wok or large, heavy frying pan over medium heat. Add the garlic and onion and stir-fry for about 5 minutes, or until the onion is golden. Stir in the garam masala, coriander, and mint. Add the chicken and cook over medium heat for 5 minutes, stirring occasionally.

2. Add the water, stir, raise the heat to high, and when the water is boiling, lower the heat to a simmer without a lid for 10 to 15 minutes, until the chicken is cooked and the sauce has thickened.

3. If you like fresh cilantro, stir in 1 tablespoon prior to serving.

Dr. Nandi's Huevos Rancheros

This is a stick-to-the-ribs breakfast I love to make with Kali and the kids on weekends.

2 TO 4 SERVINGS

1 tablespoon extra-virgin olive oil,
    plus olive oil from a spray
¼ cup chopped onions
3 garlic cloves, minced
3 jalapeño peppers, seeded and
    diced
1 (15-ounce) can chopped tomatoes,
    low sodium preferred
Pinch of sea salt

Pinch of chili powder
4 large eggs
4 corn tortillas
Beans, black or pinto
Sour cream or crumbled queso
    blanco or other white crumbly
    cheese
1 avocado, pitted and sliced

1. Heat the oil in a medium skillet over medium heat.

2. Add the onions, garlic, jalapeños, tomatoes, salt, and chili powder. Bring the sauce to a boil. Reduce the heat and let simmer for about 10 minutes.

3. Spray a second pan with olive oil and lightly fry the eggs for a few minutes, or until the egg yolks are set but still slightly undercooked.

4. Spray a third frying pan with olive oil and lightly heat the tortillas for about 30 seconds per side.

5. Place each tortilla on a plate with a serving of beans and an egg, and cover with the sauce. The sauce will cook the top of the egg. Put a dollop of sour cream on top and several slices of avocado. Serve hot.

Dr. Nandi's Egg and Avocado Toast

Fast serious nutrition on those days you need to fuel up and get out the door. Good fats and protein abound in this toast.

2 TO 4 SERVINGS

1 teaspoon olive oil

4 large eggs

1 ripe avocado, mashed

4 (1-ounce) slices hearty whole grain bread, toasted

¼ teaspoon kosher salt

¼ teaspoon freshly ground black pepper

Cherry tomatoes, for serving

1. Heat the oil in a large nonstick skillet over medium heat; swirl to coat.

2. Crack the eggs into the skillet; cook for 2 minutes. Cover and cook for 2 minutes more, or until the desired degree of doneness.

3. Spread one-quarter of the mashed avocado evenly over each toast slice. Top each toast slice with 1 fried egg. Sprinkle the eggs with salt and pepper. Serve with cherry tomatoes.

Dr. Nandi's Go-To Green Tea and Berry Smoothie

Flush out your cells with green tea and colorful berries, while getting protein from the milk and natural energy from the complex carbs in fruit and honey.

2 SERVINGS

1 cup milk
1 cup frozen organic raspberries
1 cup frozen organic blueberries
⅓ cup green tea

1 tablespoon honey
Chopped fresh mint, for garnish
Lime slices, for garnish

Blend the milk, raspberries, blueberries, tea, and honey and garnish with mint and lime. The frozen fruits give this cool smoothie its chill.

Dr. Nandi's Butternut Squash Tacos

Fall is the time to celebrate all things gourd, from pumpkins on the steps to butternut soup steaming on the table. Did you know squash makes a wonderful taco? Now you do.

4 SERVINGS

SALSA

2 garlic cloves, diced

1 jalapeño pepper, seeded and diced

¼ cup sliced white onions

1 medium tomato, seeded and diced, or 1 cup chopped tomatoes

½ ripe avocado, pitted and diced

3 tablespoons chopped fresh cilantro

¼ teaspoon salt

Freshly ground black pepper

TACOS

4 cups peeled, diced (½ inch) butternut squash

3 to 4 small dried red chile peppers

2 garlic cloves, unpeeled, smashed, and left whole

1 tablespoon extra-virgin olive oil

¾ teaspoon dried oregano, preferably Mexican

½ teaspoon salt

¼ teaspoon whole cumin seeds

2 cups cooked and drained pinto beans (see Tip 1)

½ teaspoon ground toasted cumin seeds (see Tip 2)

½ teaspoon chili powder

Freshly ground black pepper

8 (6-inch) corn tortillas

½ cup fresh cilantro leaves

½ cup finely shredded and chopped red or green cabbage

8 teaspoons crumbled queso fresco or feta cheese

TO MAKE THE SALSA

1. Toast the diced garlic, jalapeño, and onions in a dry medium skillet over medium heat, turning occasionally, until browned, fragrant, and soft, 5 to 7 minutes.

2. Combine the garlic, jalapeño, onions, tomato, and avocado in a blender or food processor. Process until smooth. Stir in the cilantro, salt, and black pepper. Set aside for topping the tacos.

TO MAKE THE TACOS

1. Preheat the oven to 400°F.

2. In a medium bowl, combine the butternut squash, chiles, smashed garlic, oil, ½ teaspoon of the oregano, ¼ teaspoon of the salt, and the whole cumin seeds; toss to coat. Arrange on a baking sheet in a single layer. Bake until soft and beginning to brown, 20 to 25 minutes.

3. Meanwhile, combine the beans in a small saucepan with the remaining ¼ teaspoon oregano, the remaining ¼ teaspoon salt, the ground cumin, chili powder, and black pepper. Heat over medium-low heat for about 10 minutes.

4. Warm the tortillas one at a time in a large dry cast-iron (or similar heavy) skillet over medium heat until soft and pliable. Wrap in a clean towel to keep warm as you go. Spoon ¼ cup of the warm beans into each tortilla; divide the roasted squash evenly among the tacos and top each with cilantro, cabbage, 2 tablespoons of the salsa, and the cheese. (Refrigerate the remaining salsa for up to 2 days.)

Tip 1: *Canned beans add speed and convenience to meal preparation. Drain the beans in a colander before using in a dish.*

Tip 2: *Put the whole cumin seeds in a small frying pan over medium-high heat. After the seeds become fragrant, remove from the heat, cool, and grind for the dish.*

Nandi #Tribe's Power Kale Bowtie Pasta Salad

Kale seemed to come upon us out of nowhere, and now it's everywhere. Few foods are healthier. If you don't like the flavor, try baby kale. It's more expensive but milder. Spinach is a viable substitute; season the dish as necessary, as spinach is one of the mildest of all greens.

6 SERVINGS

6 tablespoons light mayonnaise

⅓ cup grated Parmesan cheese

3 tablespoons lemon juice

1 tablespoon Dijon mustard

1 tablespoon extra-virgin
olive oil

1 garlic clove, peeled and crushed

½ teaspoon salt

½ teaspoon pepper

1 pound bowtie pasta (we also like
quinoa pasta)

1 large bunch kale, stemmed and
chopped

8 medium radishes, quartered

1 cup halved grape tomatoes

1 red onion, sliced into rings

1 to 2 cucumbers, washed and
chopped

1. Blend or whisk the mayonnaise, Parmesan, lemon juice, mustard, oil, garlic, salt, and pepper.

2. Bring a large saucepan of water to a boil, add salt to the cooking water, and cook the pasta according to the package instructions.

3. Mix the pasta, kale, radishes, tomatoes, onion, and cucumbers; toss in the dressing, and serve.

Dr. Nandi's Pineapple-Grilled Shrimp Salad

If you've ever gone tropical, you know that pineapple and shrimp are magnificent partners.

4 SERVINGS

MARINADE

2 tablespoons extra-virgin olive oil

2 tablespoons high-quality tequila

1 teaspoon agave nectar or honey

2 tablespoons low-sodium soy sauce

1 teaspoon ground cumin

1 teaspoon red pepper flakes

1 pound large shrimp, peeled and deveined

2 cups pineapple chunks

DRESSING

2 tablespoons extra-virgin olive oil

1 teaspoon high-quality tequila

2 teaspoons low-sodium soy sauce

2 tablespoons fresh orange juice

2 tablespoons fresh lime juice

½ teaspoon ground cumin

½ teaspoon red pepper flakes

6 cups dark leafy mixed greens

½ cup thinly sliced roasted red peppers

¼ cup toasted pine nuts

TO MAKE THE MARINADE

1. Whisk the oil, tequila, agave nectar, soy sauce, cumin, and red pepper flakes in a medium bowl. Add the shrimp and pineapple. Toss to coat the shrimp and marinate in the refrigerator for 30 minutes.

2. Remove the shrimp from the marinade. Grill the shrimp and pineapple or sauté in a large skillet over medium heat until the shrimp turns light pink and curls in on itself.

TO MAKE THE DRESSING

Whisk the oil, tequila, soy sauce, orange juice, lime juice, cumin, and red pepper flakes in a small bowl. Add the mixed greens and red peppers. Toss gently to combine. Top with the shrimp, pineapple, and pine nuts.

Dr. Nandi's Ginger Sesame Salmon

Fish is a brain food, full of omega fatty acids, and few of us eat enough of it. Large ocean fish carry heavy metals, so you should limit your intake to once or twice a week (that includes all those tuna sandwiches). Small fish such as mackerel and sardines do not carry the pollution the large fish do. Try to work the little guys into your diet, and once or twice a week, partake in a fillet like this one.

4 SERVINGS

MARINADE
¼ cup olive oil
2 tablespoons low-sodium soy sauce
2 tablespoons rice vinegar
2 tablespoons sesame oil
2 tablespoons brown sugar

2 garlic cloves, minced
1 tablespoon grated fresh ginger
1 tablespoon sesame seeds
4 green onions, thinly sliced

4 salmon fillets (the size should meet the appetites)

1. In a medium bowl, whisk the olive oil, soy sauce, vinegar, sesame oil, sugar, garlic, ginger, sesame seeds, and green onions until well combined.

2. Place the salmon in a shallow bowl, pour the marinade over the salmon, and cover the dish. Place in the refrigerator and marinate for at least 30 minutes to overnight.

3. Remove the salmon from the marinade. Grill or sauté the salmon for 3 to 5 minutes per side, or until the salmon is flaky in the center.

A BIT OF INFO ON KING SALMON

King salmon comes from Southeast Alaska, where they are allowed to troll (different than trawl) for salmon. The trollers are usually small boats, up to forty feet in length. They lower weighted hooks into the water and then troll, or motor slowly, usually around three knots, through the water and wait until the salmon hit the unbaited hooks. The salmon come aboard individually rather than being net caught. They are handled carefully and iced to preserve quality. Trawl-caught king salmon are usually better quality than net-caught because of the method of fishing and handling.

Aloo Gobi

This is another favorite dish from my birth country. It is full of the health and longevity-giving antioxidants of our spices: curry, turmeric, and cumin.

4 TO 6 SERVINGS

3 tablespoons olive oil, plus more as needed

1 teaspoon cumin seeds

1 large potato, peeled and cut into chunks

1 large head cauliflower, cut into chunks

1 teaspoon salt, or to taste

1 tablespoon ground turmeric

2 teaspoons ground cumin

2 teaspoons curry powder

¼ teaspoon cayenne pepper, or to taste

1 cup organic frozen peas

1 teaspoon granulated sugar

Cilantro, for garnish

1. In a large skillet with a cover, heat the oil over medium heat and brown the cumin seeds for a minute. Add the potato and cauliflower, stirring often, and cook for about 5 minutes.

2. Add the salt, turmeric, cumin, curry powder, and cayenne. Stir and coat the cauliflower and potato with the spices.

3. Sauté for another few minutes, adding a bit more oil or water if needed. Add 1 cup of water and stir to coat evenly.

4. Cover and cook over medium heat, stirring occasionally, for about 15 minutes. After the potatoes and cauliflower are soft, add the peas and sugar and cook for about 5 minutes, or until the peas are heated through. Garnish with cilantro and serve.

Dr. Nandi's Chicken Curry II

In this version of chicken curry, Kali and I add coconut milk and lots of fixings for the kids to sprinkle atop their meal.

4 SERVINGS

1 tablespoon olive oil

1 tablespoon unsalted butter

3 garlic cloves, crushed

1 medium onion, finely chopped

2 tablespoons garam masala

1 teaspoon ground coriander

½ teaspoon dried mint

1½ pounds boneless, skinless chicken breast, diced

1 cup coconut milk

OPTIONAL GARNISHES

Chopped fresh cilantro

¼ cup raisins

½ cup shredded unsweetened coconut

½ cup slivered almonds

2 hard-boiled eggs, chopped

1. Heat the oil and butter in a wok or large, heavy frying pan. Add the garlic and onion and stir-fry for about 5 minutes, until the onion is golden.

2. Stir in the garam masala, coriander, and mint. Add the chicken and cook over medium heat for 5 minutes, stirring occasionally.

3. Add the coconut milk, stir, and simmer without a lid for 10 to 15 minutes, until the chicken is cooked and the sauce has thickened. If you like cilantro, stir in 1 tablespoon prior to serving. Serve with optional garnishes.

Dal

Dal is life for huge numbers of people in the world. Imagine what it can do for you!

4 SERVINGS

1 tablespoon olive oil

1 teaspoon cumin seeds

1 small onion, diced

1 teaspoon ground cumin

1 teaspoon ground turmeric

1 teaspoon curry powder

1 teaspoon garam masala

1 teaspoon salt

½ teaspoon cayenne pepper, or to taste

1 large bay leaf, or 2 small

1 cup masoor dal (red lentils)

4 cups water

Chopped fresh cilantro, for garnish (optional)

1 green chile, diced, for garnish (optional)

1. In a medium saucepan, heat the oil and sauté the cumin seeds and onion. Once the onion becomes translucent, about 2 minutes, add the ground cumin, turmeric, curry powder, garam masala, salt, cayenne, and bay leaf. Cook for about 1 minute, stirring often, until the spices become aromatic.

2. Add the dal and stir to coat with the spices. Add the water to the saucepan. Bring to a boil, then reduce the heat, cover, and cook for about 30 minutes. Remove and discard the bay leaf. Garnish with the cilantro and green chile, if desired, and serve.

Dr. Nandi's Thai Cabbage Leaf Wraps with Chicken

This is the Nandi family take on a beloved Thai dish.

4 SERVINGS

1 cup water

¾ cup sliced red onions

1 pound ground organic chicken breast

3 tablespoons finely chopped fresh mint

2 tablespoons finely chopped fresh cilantro

3 tablespoons fresh lime juice

4 teaspoons Thai fish sauce

¼ to ½ teaspoon crushed red pepper flakes

16 organic napa (Chinese) cabbage leaves (about 1 head)

Lime wedges (optional)

1. Heat the water in a nonstick skillet over medium-high heat. Add the onions and chicken to the skillet. Cook for 5 minutes, stirring to break up the chicken, or until the chicken is cooked through. Drain. Return the chicken mixture to the skillet over medium heat; stir in the mint, cilantro, lime juice, fish sauce, and red pepper flakes. Mix until heated through.

2. Spoon about 3 tablespoons of the chicken mixture onto each cabbage leaf. Roll the leaf over the chicken mixture, fold over the long sides of the leaf, and continue to roll the leaf as you would to make a burrito. Serve with lime wedges, if desired.

Dr. Nandi's Veggie Hummus Club Sandwich

Delicious and mobile, this sandwich fits the on-the-go Nandi #healthhero life to a tee.

4 SERVINGS

3 tablespoons plain fat-free yogurt

2 tablespoons water

1 tablespoon lemon juice

1 tablespoon tahini

½ teaspoon ground cumin

¼ teaspoon salt

2 garlic cloves, peeled

1 (15-ounce) can chickpeas, rinsed and drained

12 slices whole wheat or gluten-free bread

2 cups shredded Bibb lettuce

8 slices tomato

4 slices red onion

1 cup sliced cucumber

4 cups alfalfa sprouts

1. Combine the yogurt, water, lemon juice, tahini, cumin, salt, garlic, and chickpeas in a food processor; process until smooth.

2. Spread 2 tablespoons hummus over 1 bread slice; top with ½ cup lettuce, 2 tomato slices, 1 onion slice, 1 bread slice, ¼ cup sliced cucumber, 1 cup sprouts, and 1 bread slice.

3. Cut the sandwich diagonally into quarters; secure with wooden picks.

4. Repeat the procedure with the remaining ingredients.

Dr. Nandi's Freekeh Burger

Freekeh is ground durum wheat that's roasted and rubbed, creating an incomparable flavor in North African and Mediterranean cuisines. This is exotic fun food exploration for your #tribe.

4 TO 6 SERVINGS

3 cups cooked organic pinto beans

1 cup cracked freekeh

5 cloves garlic, minced

½ cup shredded carrots

½ cup sliced green onions

2 tablespoons za'atar

2 teaspoons ground cumin

Salt and freshly ground black pepper, to taste

2 large eggs, lightly beaten

2 tablespoons olive oil, plus more as needed

2 large onions, thinly sliced

1 tablespoon harissa

8 hamburger buns

Baby spinach leaves, for serving

1. Preheat the oven to 350°F. Line a baking sheet with parchment paper. Place the beans in a large bowl and mash them lightly.

2. Stir in the freekeh, garlic, carrots, and green onions. Add the za'atar 1 teaspoon at a time (taste the mixture to find the correct amount for your liking).

3. Stir in the cumin, salt, and pepper, then fold in the eggs. Form the mixture into 8 large patties.

4. Put the patties on the baking sheet. Brush the tops of the patties with oil and bake for about 25 minutes (you want them golden and slightly crispy on the edges).

5. While the burgers are in the oven, heat 2 tablespoons oil in a large skillet over medium heat. Add the onions and a pinch of salt; cook for 8 to 10 minutes. Stir in the harissa slowly and keep adding to taste.

6. To make the burgers, place each patty on a bun and top with the onions, smoky garlic aioli (recipe below), and spinach leaves.

SMOKY GARLIC AIOLI

1 teaspoon cumin seeds

1 teaspoon coriander seeds

1 cup organic mayonnaise

4 tablespoons extra-virgin olive oil

4 teaspoons fresh lemon juice

1 tablespoon smoked paprika

2 to 3 garlic cloves, pressed

Salt and freshly ground black pepper, to taste

1. Toast the cumin seeds and coriander seeds in a small dry skillet over medium-high heat, about 1½ minutes. Cool.

2. Finely grind the toasted seeds. Put them into a small bowl and whisk in the mayonnaise, oil, lemon juice, paprika, and garlic. Season the aioli with salt and pepper.

Dr. Nandi's Tomato and Nectarine Salad

So easy and fresh, it's ready in minutes and has great nutritional power.

4 SERVINGS

3 tablespoons balsamic vinegar
1 teaspoon honey
4 tomatoes
3 nectarines
1 ball fresh mozzarella
¾ cup fresh basil leaves

Extra-virgin organic olive oil (you
    want to have enough to drizzle
    over the salad)
Salt and freshly ground black pep-
    per, to taste

1. In a small saucepan, heat the vinegar and honey over medium heat until the mixture reaches a syrupy consistency.

2. Slice the tomatoes, nectarines, and mozzarella in wedges of approximately the same size and arrange them on a platter with the basil leaves.

3. Drizzle the oil over the top and sprinkle with salt and pepper.

4. Drizzle the balsamic-honey mixture around the edge of the platter and over the salad. Serve and enjoy!

Dr. Nandi's Sake and Udon Noodle Salmon

This dish is full of omega fatty acids in the sesame and salmon. Your brain and nervous system will thank you.

4 SERVINGS

1 tablespoon unsalted butter

¼ cup sliced shallots

2 teaspoons minced fresh ginger

½ cup sake

2½ cups hot water

1 tablespoon miso paste

1 (14-ounce) can chicken or vegetable broth

1 cup sliced shiitake or cremini mushrooms

½ cup sliced green onions

½ cup julienned carrots

½ cup sliced green beans

4 Alaskan sockeye salmon, rinsed and cut into bite-size pieces

16 ounces cooked udon noodles

1 teaspoon sesame seeds

1. In a large skillet, heat the butter over medium heat and sauté the shallots and ginger until the shallots are softened, about 2 minutes. Add the sake and cook until the liquid is reduced by about half.

2. Add the water and miso and whisk until smooth. Stir in the broth, mushrooms, green onions, carrots, and green beans and bring to a simmer.

3. Add the fish to the broth, cook for 2 minutes, then remove the skillet from the heat and let rest for 5 minutes, until the salmon is opaque throughout. Divide the udon noodles among the bowls and add 1 cup of fish and broth to each bowl, topping with the sesame seeds. Serve piping hot.

Dr. Nandi's Shrimp Tacos

Where there are kids, there are tacos. Where there are adults, there are tacos. Everybody loves tacos. They make a perfect delivery device for getting good nutrition into small and large stomachs alike.

4 SERVINGS

2½ tablespoons olive oil

4 teaspoons fresh lime juice

¼ teaspoon ground cumin

¼ teaspoon hot smoked paprika

¼ teaspoon crushed red pepper flakes

1 pound medium shrimp, peeled and deveined

⅓ cup sliced green onions

¼ teaspoon salt

½ teaspoon grated lime zest

1 Granny Smith apple, cored and thinly sliced

1 jalapeño pepper, seeded and minced

8 (6-inch) corn tortillas

1 ounce crumbled queso fresco

1. Combine 1 tablespoon of the oil, 2 teaspoons of the lime juice, the cumin, paprika, and red pepper flakes in a small bowl.

2. Put the shrimp and spice mixture in a zip-top plastic bag and seal. Let stand for 15 minutes.

3. In the same bowl, combine the remaining 1½ tablespoons oil, the remaining 2 teaspoons lime juice, the green onions, ⅛ teaspoon of the salt, the lime zest, apple, and jalapeño and mix. Set the salsa aside.

4. Remove the shrimp from the bag and discard the marinade.

5. Heat a large grill pan over medium-high heat.

6. Sprinkle the shrimp with the remaining ⅛ teaspoon salt.

7. Arrange half the shrimp in the pan; grill for 2 minutes per side, or until pink. Remove from the pan, making sure to keep the shrimp warm. Repeat the procedure with the remaining shrimp.

8. Place 2 tortillas each on 4 plates, and divide the shrimp evenly among the tortillas. Divide the salsa evenly among the tacos, and top with the queso fresco.

Dr. Nandi's Red, White, and Blue Salad

Here is my healthy tribute to the colors of my adopted home.

4 SERVINGS

9 ounces baby spinach, torn
1 cup sliced strawberries
1 cup raspberries
1 cup blueberries
½ cup sliced almonds, toasted

⅓ cup chopped basil
1 avocado, pitted and chopped
4 ounces blue cheese, crumbled
Strawberry or raspberry balsamic
    vinegar, for drizzling

1. Divide the baby spinach among 4 plates, then top with the berries, almonds, basil, and avocado.

2. Sprinkle with the blue cheese, then drizzle with vinegar to taste. It really is that simple!

chapter three

THE #HEALTHHERO MOVEMENT PLAN

Everything old *is* new again! Consider this headline on National Public Radio's *Morning Edition* in 2010: "100 Years Ago, Exercise Was Blended Into Daily Life." Our grandparents utilized two to three times as many calories a day as we do. Couple that with how they used their bodies to create day-to-day life and you have ancestral #healthheroes that you didn't even know existed.

In the NPR piece, Adrian Bauman, a professor of public health and epidemiology at the University of Sydney, said it best: "We don't expend energy doing anything. We've actually engineered regular daily physical activity out of our lives." He went on to describe the modern life as walking to the car, driving to the office, sitting for eight hours, walking back to the car, and then traveling home to sit on the couch. Imagine—with driverless cars, we won't even have to turn the wheel!

Ouch! Have we really fallen that far?

The answer is yes, and that's another reason the idea of the #healthhero was born. When we talk about health, we are actually talking about how you live your life, and the best way to improve everything is *to move.*

Everything, you say? Well, yes. Without movement, the #healthhero is without a huge tool in the fight against disease and early death. Without movement, brain function suffers and mood disorders abound. Without movement, blood flow is restricted and certain organs receive less than optimal support. Joints and hinges don't get worked and stiffen up. Movement literally has an impact on every function and process of the body, a fact that Bernarr Macfadden, a pioneer in the physical fitness movement, touted more than a hundred years ago. Macfadden believed external flexibility signaled, in part, inner flexibility, both physical and mental. Without movement, it is hard to be a hero of any kind.

That's what the #healthhero must adopt today. Life *is* exercise and you don't need to spend one cent to reach your goals. The magic number is thirty minutes a day.

You don't need to spend money on a gym or personal trainer. You don't need to jump into a training program that would make Michael Phelps dizzy. What you need to do is learn how to move around inside your life in a way that is pleasing, fun, and healthy for you. Everything you do is an opportunity to burn calories, and every object around you is a potential weight to lift or ball to throw. Sidewalks are for walking, so do so, as often as possible. Beat that batter by hand instead of using the mixer, wash your own car instead of going to the car wash on the way home from work.

Life! Life is your workout and you will always have time for it, unlike the three hours it takes to get in and out of a gym. I also see well-meaning patients who love spending those hours and more working out diligently. However, there is a fine line between the right amount of exercise and the dangers of overexercising.

Look at Robert, my patient who loved to work out. He was experienced, knowing the importance of lifting weights and aerobic training.

He loved to run and bike. "I feel so refreshed, energetic, and revitalized when I work out!" he said.

He was always looking for a challenge, so CrossFit became his next challenge to master. His friends raved about the regimen and told him how amazing it felt. So away Robert went, into the studio, filled with excitement.

Upon registering, he filled out all the forms and disclaimers, signing them quickly. He was ready to start this adventure now! So he stepped into a space, raw in appearance, with vehicle tires and kettlebells. *Wow,* he thought. *This is gonna be great.* So he began to work out every day, rarely missing. He continued to push himself to achieve greater goals, often pushing his body to its limit.

On a rainy Saturday, Robert was at the CrossFit gym. He was determined to give his best performance yet! He felt great and began with passion. As his workout continued, he felt a little different than he had before. He had more pain in his muscles and felt as if he would vomit. He felt light-headed and stumbled to the bathroom. Robert would recall that his urine was the color of blood.

He had difficulty moving and asked the staff of the facility for help. They too were alarmed and unsure what to do. Why was this muscular, vibrant man, a stud, suddenly stumbling, unable to maintain his balance, and appearing ill? They called 911 asking for help. Scared and unsure, they wanted Robert to be taken to the hospital.

In the emergency room, Robert was confused, not quite sure what was happening. The doctors asked his friend, who had accompanied him to the hospital, what was going on. Nothing out of the ordinary, his friend recalled. James was a little scared, never having seen his workout buddy Robert look like this. He watched as the doctors and nurses examined and treated Robert. Blood tests were ordered and multiple vials of blood were sent to the lab. IVs were started and fluids were given to this wounded workout warrior.

James asked the medical team for answers. Why was his friend urinating blood? Why was his blood pressure so low? Why was his heart rate so high? Was Robert going to be okay? The nurse reassured him, telling him that Robert was going to be tested so they could understand what was going on. Minutes became hours, and finally the doctor came into the small room to speak with Robert and James. His heart racing, James feared the worst. Robert wasn't getting better. What was going to happen next?

Rhabdomyolysis: That's what the doctor said. James couldn't even pronounce it, let alone understand what the word meant. The doctor said that Robert's muscles were damaged and the damage had spilled into his blood. She felt that he would be okay but recommended admission to the intensive care unit for more treatment. His intense CrossFit workout had resulted in this damage, which could potentially be very serious, even life-threatening.

The ICU! James's worst fears had come true. He waited for Robert's parents, who were gone for the weekend.

In the ICU, the nurses and doctors treated Robert with the utmost care, watching his vital signs and taking daily blood tests. They were concerned that his kidneys were damaged and might fail. He was placed on dialysis to help his kidneys filter the toxins. His family stayed in the hospital day and night. They couldn't believe this was happening! Their son, strong and healthy, was battling to save his organs. After days of treatment, Robert was then transferred to the general medical floor. He was becoming his old self, cheerful and upbeat.

Little did Robert realize that starting a fitness program could nearly cost him his life. Exercise was his passion. Following every fad, always pursuing the newest regimen, was his modus operandi. Several weeks after his discharge from the hospital, he read the papers he had signed at the CrossFit gym. He saw the word *rhabdomyolysis* in the paperwork; the boilerplate in the contract mentioned that this might be a complication of this workout. He wished that he had understood the meaning of that word earlier.

Fitness is a great tool for a healthy life. However, as in Robert's case, not understanding what types of fitness are appropriate and not understanding the risks may be really detrimental to your health.

So to begin, we should ask ourselves, "Why am I exercising? Why am I doing this activity? Is it to become healthier, or do I just want to look better? Do I want to do it because it's the cool new trend?" Not understanding *why* you should move and exercise can lead to problems in your health and well-being. A #healthhero's movement is determined by his or her goals of wellness and true health rather than a six-pack and swelling biceps.

Endorphin release provides a high, albeit a natural one, and individuals overexercise looking for that rush. Obsessive personalities are forever upping the hours they dedicate to fitness, and gyms nationwide are filled with people with eating disorders, frantically pedaling away the calories of their cup of frozen yogurt. Be reasonable. Find the balance and you'll tap into a wellspring of energy, health, and longevity.

We all know that exercise is helpful to us. But how is it helpful? What does this movement do for us? Let's start with the physical benefits, not the sculpted bodies that are defined as "beautiful." The stuff on the inside is what I'm talking about.

My patient Roberta understood this fact. She had gained sixty pounds in the past several years.

"It just crept up on me, Doc, and all of a sudden, I was the heaviest I had ever been," she told me.

With her weight gain came relentless knee and hip pain, often keeping her up at night. Ibuprofen became her BFF, and she used this drug to help her move better and keep the pain at bay. Using up to six pills of ibuprofen a day, Roberta could find some relief, allowing her to sleep a few hours.

However, one night she suddenly had stomach pain, so severe that she went to the hospital, worrying if she was having a heart attack. The emergency department excluded any heart problems with blood testing, an EKG, and a heart ultrasound. I was called to help determine the reason for her symptoms. When I examined Roberta, she had exquisite tenderness in her left upper abdomen. Concerned about what could be causing her distress, I performed an upper endoscopy, in which I inserted a flexible lighted scope into her stomach.

I found a large ulcer there and irritation of her esophagus. I began treating the ulcer and Roberta's stomach pain gradually decreased; the problem, though, became more complicated. With her joint pain, she needed help. Her medicines for the joint pain had caused a big problem in her stomach and esophagus. I asked Roberta to start slowly and follow a #healthhero movement guide and a #healthhero diet.

My patient worked diligently to exercise thirty minutes per day for several months. Her diet improved dramatically, and Roberta felt increased energy and decreased pain. Those joints needed to move! Her weight decreased significantly, twenty pounds in three months. Her pain was controlled and she felt empowered.

Roberta's story is not unique. One of the main benefits of movement and exercise is weight control. Even a few minutes a day helps. Exercise also moves the hinges and joints, keeping them "greased," so to speak. For when it comes to the body, the saying "use it or lose it" is absolutely true. Don't worry about the gym: Life provides plenty of exercise for most individuals. Let me explain what I mean.

Instead of taking the elevator, take the stairs. Park as far away from the entrance of the store as you can. Take a bike to work instead of the car. Carry your own groceries. Garden. Work in the yard. If you sit all day, stand up every hour and walk, stretch and breathe deeply for at least five minutes. Put an exercise ball in your office (if that's allowed) and stretch your back out several times a day. (Later in the chapter, there are many ideas for desk stretches to keep your blood pumping all day.) If you have trouble motivating yourself for a daily walk, add a dog to your family or ask a member of your #tribe to be your strolling partner. Sing and dance around your house, alone or with an audience to spur you on.

Use a gallon of milk as a weight and lift it ten times with one arm, ten times with the other. Repeat. Tilt your head back and look at the sky, giving your spine a nice stretch and your heart a beautiful blue view. Life is your workout, and it's free.

Your body will thank you and you will not need membership in a fancy, expensive gym. What you will receive are the benefits of movement with purpose: weight control, increased energy, and improvement in your numbers, which gauge blood pressure, blood sugar levels, and cholesterol.

In a review of ninety-three trials in the *Journal of Hypertension*, Veronique Cornelissen and Neil Smart found that exercise decreases blood pressure in individuals. Thirty minutes of moderate exercise daily will do the trick! Up to 43 percent of the US population are affected with hypertension, and almost 1 billion people worldwide suffer from this disease, so we need to stop this killer. Heart disease, congestive heart failure, and stroke are just some of the problems you can encounter. Kidney problems are also possible with uncontrolled high blood pressure. Some people even experience vision loss and sexual dysfunction. Spending a few extra minutes a day to include movement can make all the difference between life and a life of tragedy.

Jimmy came to see me with his wife. His physician asked me to help with a feeding tube. Jimmy had suffered a stroke recently and could not swallow properly, choking on food whenever he tried to swallow. He'd had hypertension for a long time but didn't control it well. He always "felt good" and didn't know that he had any problems. Despite the constant encouragement of his wife and son, he would not exercise, often spending the weekends parked on the couch. Then early one morning, he was slurring his speech and could not move well.

His wife, Roberta, rushed him to the hospital. Jimmy was terrified and so was his family. He couldn't understand what was happening. With the help of blood tests and CT scans and MRIs, he was diagnosed with a stroke. He was admitted to the hospital and treated with physical and occupational therapy. Jimmy worked hard and listened to everything the therapists asked him to do. His speech slowly improved and he was able to walk with a cane.

However, his swallowing did not get significantly better. He was not able to take in the food he needed to maintain enough nutrition. Jimmy was very unhappy about the prospect of a tube to get his nutrition. He spent many sleepless nights thinking about the tube. I told Jimmy that the tube might be temporary and he should continue to work on his therapy. If his swallowing improved, I could easily remove the tube and he would be able to eat all the food himself! He was encouraged by this and agreed to have the procedure to place a tube into his stomach for nutrition.

Jimmy and Roberta arrived at the hospital and checked in at the receptionist. They were very nervous. I met with them, assuring them that everything would be okay. Jimmy was wheeled into the procedure area and was still nervous, but seemed less anxious than when he had entered the hospital. The anesthesiologist gave him the medication and he fell asleep very quickly. I then placed an endoscope, a long black tube, into his mouth, then down through his esophagus, and finally into his stomach. His stomach looked normal and healthy. I then located the best place to insert the tube to help Jimmy survive.

I made an incision on his abdomen; a place to insert the feeding tube. The tube was long and the procedure went smoothly. At the end of the surgery, there was a tube outside Jimmy's body, entering the stomach, in which he and his family could place food and medicines.

When he awoke, Jimmy had mild pain but was doing well. He wanted to see the tube, so I showed him. He was emotional as the reality of the situation crept into his brain. His wife and I reassured him, reminding him that it might be temporary. Our reassurances weren't enough and Jimmy couldn't hold back the tears. I tried to console him, with little success.

What if Jimmy had done what I'm asking you to do now? What if he had listened to his family? What if he had spent a few minutes every day, making simple decisions with his fork and moving with purpose? Instead of weekends on the couch, watching athletes move with precision, he could walk, bike, garden, or just do some chores around the house. Although these decisions are simple, becoming a #healthhero involves making such decisions every day. The rewards are tremendous, for yourself and your family. If only Jimmy had made #healthhero decisions, the course of his life would have been dramatically different.

In addition to having hypertension, Jimmy suffered from another killer: obesity. Obesity is a worldwide epidemic reaching crisis proportions and draining health-care resources. Today nearly 2.1 billion people are obese, with the numbers doubling in the last two decades. As you may know, obesity has been associated with many health risks. Hypertension and stroke are more likely. Many cancers occur with increasing obesity. Obese patients are significantly more likely to develop diabetes, which has its own devastating complications. Gallbladder problems are more prevalent, and being obese increases osteoarthritis and gout as well.

To understand the spread of obesity, let us examine a five-year period between 1995 and 2000. The National Institutes of Health cite a 36 percent rise in health-care spending due to obesity. In England, 1 in

4 adults is obese. The World Health Organization calls this "globesity," and it is spreading like wildfire. In 1995, there were an estimated 200 million obese adults and 18 million obese *children under five.* By the year 2000, just five short years later, the number of obese adults rose to 300 million. Contrary to popular belief, obesity is not just a first world problem. In 2000, 115 million of those obese adults were in developing countries.

Today, one-third of all Americans are classified as obese and obesity is three times more responsible for death than previously thought, according to recent research by Columbia University in New York City. Black women are the most vulnerable, with white women second. A co-author of this study, Ryan Masters, said in a statement released in 2013: "Obesity has dramatically worse health consequences than some recent reports have led us to believe."

The surgeon general of the United States estimates 300,000 deaths from obesity a year. That's more than the Vietnam War and the wars in the Middle East combined. In just two years at this pace, it will outdistance AIDS (638,000 deaths, according to the Centers for Disease Control and Prevention) as a killer.

Increased activity and exercise reduce obesity and slow weight gain. In the Nurses' Health Study II from Brigham and Women's Hospital and Harvard Medical School, 18,000 women were studied. The women who increased their activity by thirty minutes a day had less weight gain than those who didn't. Christine Friedenreich studied the effectiveness of moderate activity on weight gain and published the results in the *International Journal of Obesity.* Researchers found that at the end of a year, there was significantly decreased obesity in those who undertook moderate activity. Although this finding seems intuitive, many of us don't perform the activities that would help to prevent and treat obesity. If we spend a few minutes of our day doing the activities of a #healthhero and move more often, we can achieve our goals of health and wellness.

Along with obesity, another significant health problem involves high cholesterol. Hypercholesterolemia can affect your health significantly. Cholesterol forms deposits on the walls of your blood vessels, which can result in heart attacks and strokes, leading killers on our planet. High cholesterol can increase the risk of gallstones as well, and the arteries supplying blood to your legs and arms can also be affected by high cholesterol.

High cholesterol is often called a "silent killer" because the only way to find it is by testing the blood and its pressure. That's the first thing I did with Rosalie. Rosalie was a pleasant woman, always cheerful. She saw me periodically for troubles with acid reflux. Her blood pressure was quite often high, to which she responded that when she checked her blood pressure at home, it was always normal! Rosalie also suffered from high cholesterol. Her bad cholesterol, LDL, was high and her good cholesterol, HDL, was low. I often spoke to Rosalie about her cholesterol as well as her hypertension and her increasing weight.

She would always reply, "Doc, I'm just enjoying life!"

I was called to the hospital on a hot summer day. A patient was bleeding, with bloody bowel movements and a low blood count with decreased hemoglobin. I rushed to the hospital to find dear Rosalie, sweating, a distressed look on her face. Gone was her cheerfulness, replaced by fear and anxiety. I held her hand and let her know that her team of doctors would do everything they could to help her. Her job was not to worry and stay calm and focused.

Rosalie had been rushed to the hospital earlier after complaining of being nauseated and short of breath. Her son had been visiting her and called 911 when his mother worsened. He was concerned and unsure of what was happening to his mother, the family's pillar of strength. The ambulance came and took Rosalie to the hospital, only ten minutes away from her home. In the emergency department, Rosalie seemed slightly but not significantly improved. The doctors and nurses evaluated her, and after a few tests and an EKG, the diagnosis was made.

She was having a heart attack. Rosalie was scared. Was she going to make it? The cardiologist came and assessed her and performed a heart catheterization, in which a catheter was placed in Rosalie's groin and dye was injected into the blood vessels of her heart. She had blockages, which were treated by the expert cardiologist, likely saving her life. Then she was given medicines to thin her blood and had bloody stools.

I watched her carefully, and thankfully, she stopped bleeding and her blood count stabilized and improved over the next week. Finally I saw a glint of her smile and her upbeat personality, but she got the point of this scary episode.

"I should have taken better care of myself, Doc. You were right," she said with a sigh. All of her problems with her heart and the complications that resulted could have potentially been avoided with a few extra minutes a day of increased movement and exercise. By being her own #healthhero, Rosalie could have spent time enjoying the beautiful weather and her family. Instead, she was in a hospital bed, terrified and ill.

In 2014, Steven Mann and his colleagues reviewed thirteen trials and published their meta-analysis in *Sports Medicine*, concluding that exercise and movement help to improve cholesterol. Moderate activity and exercise benefit those like Rosalie, who suffer from high cholesterol. As an added bonus, the help with obesity and high blood pressure is also wonderful. The message to the #healthhero is loud and clear: Move with purpose to promote your health and get the benefits of this powerful preventive medicine.

IT'S NOT JUST YOUR BODY, IT'S YOUR MOOD AND YOUR THOUGHTS

So we have spoken of physical illness, of hypertension, obesity, and hypercholesterolemia. What about emotional and psychological wellness? Mental health is also critical. How do increased movement and exercise help your mood? Exercise and movement with purpose is an amazing remedy for your mood and mental health. With the global cost of mental health at over $2.5 trillion, we need help with these devastating illnesses. Movement raises endorphins, serotonin, and dopamine, those feel-good chemicals, but as more blood is pumped into the brain, this literally stops rumination and circular stressful thoughts, according to a study from the University of California, San Francisco, in 2010. In addition to the mood-stabilizing factors of exercise on the brain, movement has a huge impact on sending blood to the brain to enhance learning, according to German researchers.

They divided a group of high school students in half. One group did ten minutes of varied exercise before taking a test; the other half didn't. Guess who scored higher? You probably guessed right, and if you are a parent, you might now have a deeper understanding of why kids need exercise and play.

Rebecca visited my office in the fall. She was suffering from constipation and nausea. Often bloated and uncomfortable, she didn't know what her next step should be. I saw this young lady and asked her about any medications she was taking.

"Oh, I started this antidepressant a few weeks ago," she told me.

She then told me that her problems didn't really start until after she had started taking her antidepressant. Rebecca had suffered an injury while she was running and couldn't do her favorite activity. Running was peaceful for her and she felt free. She had suffered with periods of depressed mood throughout her life, but always seemed to snap out of it.

Rebecca's primary care doctor saw the signs of persistent depression on one of her visits and gave Rebecca a prescription for an antidepressant. It was a quick visit, Rebecca recalled. I told her that nausea and constipation are well-known side effects of antidepressants.

Although she was an avid runner, my patient didn't realize the health benefits of exercise, especially mental health. An injury to her knee had caused Rebecca to stop running. The absence of that movement in Rebecca's life depressed her mood and her body systems. "Have you ever tried yoga? How about swimming?" I asked.

She promised to ask her sports medicine doctor and let me know.

Several weeks later I saw Rebecca again. Her constipation and nausea had disappeared! Her antidepressants were also history. Getting off antidepressants is not right for everyone, but the point is, exercising will help you feel calmer and better. She took my advice and became active. With the blessing of her sports medicine doctor, she was practicing yoga several times a week and felt much better. She still had some feelings of depression, but these feelings did not leave her incapacitated. Rebecca had found the #healthhero inside her. By adopting a new method of movement, she was able to say good-bye to the pills that gave her gastrointestinal problems while preserving her mental health.

Rebecca is among the millions of people worldwide who have discovered the magic of regular exercise: It helps mild to moderate depression, and in fact may be as effective as many antidepressants! Multiple studies going back as far as 1981 have shown the effectiveness of exercise on mood and mental health. The *Archives of Internal Medicine* published a trial in which a group of men and women were studied. A third took an antidepressant, a third participated in regular exercise, and a third did both. At the end of the study, the majority of people in all three groups could not be classified as having depression! In fact, the exercise had a longer-lasting effect than the medications, the study showed. Simply amazing! The movement of the #healthhero can indeed heal the body and the mind.

So you may be asking, Just how does exercise affect mental health? Well, #healthhero movement can increase the *growth* of neurons and decrease inflammation, all helping your brain function. Exercise releases endorphins, chemicals that can elevate your spirit and mood. Also, movement distracts you, allowing you some time to reflect and sort out negative and ruminative thoughts. #Healthheroes who move also have improved sleep, leading to alert, healthy minds and well-being. They have decreased stress and a more optimistic view of themselves. All these factors help #healthheroes improve their mental health and overall wellness.

Millions suffer from anxiety every day worldwide, with an estimated one in thirteen struggling with this condition. According to the Anxiety and Depression Association of America (ADAA), there are 40 million American adults affected by anxiety disorders! These disorders can be crippling and take over the lives of patients, keeping them from thriving, from achieving their wellness goals, their life goals. Anxiety isolates the individual and affects every part of his or her life, leading to such physical problems as gastrointestinal symptoms, increased heart rate, and hyperventilation. Some anxiety even ends in suicide.

It was a lovely fall day in the heart of the Midwest; the leaves had just changed to a beautiful array of orange and yellow. I'd just finished speaking to an appreciative group regarding the epidemic of suicide in this country, including its risk factors. This was where I met Ronald's parents, who told me his tragic story. Ronald, or Junior as they called him, was a good kid. He never really got in any trouble as a young child. As

PARTHA'S RX

1. #Healthheroes incorporate movement into their daily lives. It's not necessary to join a fancy gym or an expensive class. Find your favorite activities and incorporate them into your life. Take a bike to work, garden, or take the stairs instead of the elevators.

2. Before participating in a new health regimen, the true #healthhero does research and asks his or her health-care provider. Often, injury and illness can result without the proper consultation.

3. A #healthhero knows why he or she is exercising. Knowing the reason for the activity will help motivation and dedication, ensuring success. Movement is for increased well-being, not just beautifully sculpted bodies.

4. The movement and exercise of the #healthhero can improve mental health. In fact, exercise can be as effective as some antidepressants in treating mild to moderate depression!

he grew older and entered middle and high school, he began to have difficulty dealing with symptoms of anxiety and depression.

Junior found himself paralyzed in social situations, whether it was a football game or a presentation. He had few friends and his parents struggled to help him cope with his problems. Ronald saw multiple psychiatrists and therapists. Although these professionals helped him, Ronald didn't like the way the drugs they prescribed made him feel. Besides his problems at school, some of his classmates were cruel to him in person and on social media. Junior felt that he had no escape and that the world around him was collapsing.

The pressure in Ronald's mind was unbearable, and he took his life. His parents were devastated. They later found that Junior had stopped taking his medications, likely frustrated by the side effects he was experiencing. I gave Ronald's parents my condolences and asked them if he had participated in any sports or activities. They stated he had not. What about physical activity? I asked. Not much, they answered.

Movement with purpose and exercise help with the treatment of anxiety. Moving like a #healthhero can decrease stress and anxiety, increasing endorphins and improving well-being. In *Depression and Anxiety*, Jasper Smits and his fellow researchers reported their findings from a study of the intervention of exercise on anxiety. With two weeks of exercise intervention, all participants noted a decrease in anxiety levels. These conclusions were similar to those in an article Matthew Herring and his colleagues published in the 2010 *Archives of Internal Medicine*. Here, the authors did a meta-analysis of forty trials in which exercise was utilized to help with anxiety.[1] They found that movement did indeed significantly alleviate the symptoms of anxiety.

The #healthhero movement techniques treat multiple conditions, but what about preventing some of these problems to begin with? Can exercise actually stop problems before they begin? Will we ward off disease and illness with our notion of movement with purpose? The entire field of medicine is moving toward prevention. It must, given the huge drain on the planet's resources and rapidly escalating prices. A #healthhero understands the whole picture of purpose, people, planet, and, alas, pocketbook. Techniques to combat disease before it begins are being rewarded throughout our planet.

Researcher Huseyin Naci found that exercise was equivalent to medication treatment in the prevention of diabetes and published the findings in *BMJ* (*British Medical Journal*). Imagine this benefit without the side effects of the drugs and the cost of the medications. No constipation. No sexual dysfunction. No pills to irritate the esophagus. With a decrease in obesity resulting from the movement of the #healthhero, we can prevent diseases such as those dreadful killers hypertension and heart disease.

What about cancer? Can we decrease the risk of cancer with movement and exercise? There is strong proof that breast, colon, and endometrial cancer can be reduced by 35 percent through movement. Now more evidence has been published in *JAMA* (*Journal of the American Medical Association*) showing that we can decrease the risk of thirteen cancers with exercise![2] This is simply amazing news. We can avoid the development of deadly diseases simply by walking or jogging. Countless lives and billions of dollars can be saved if more follow the motto of the #healthhero and move with purpose.

Arthritic conditions cost $65 billion per year and have patients seeing their health-care providers 44 million times per year. Some 750,000 hospitalizations result from these diseases. One of the main prevention techniques that the Arthritis Foundation recommends is exercise, along with weight control. Movement, while painful at times, increases the mobility of an arthritic joint, and weight loss eases the load it must carry.

My mother often spoke of my great-grandmother, who was healthy until she passed away peacefully in her late nineties. Thakuma (grandmother), as my mom referred to this beautiful woman, was a #healthhero. As a child in India and later as an adolescent in the United States, I would hear stories of Thakuma. Always moving, this lady seldom sat for any prolonged time. She walked everywhere and always moved with purpose. Thakuma did not suffer from any diseases and thrived throughout her life.

Thakuma is like my nurse Mary, another incredible #healthhero and a healer. She worked with her patients until her early eighties. Mary was rarely idle. She would walk during her breaks and helped her co-workers with a smile. She took no pills and had no chronic diseases. She was able to make the most of her life. Not only did these ladies not suffer from disease, but they worked actively to prevent it from attacking their bodies. While others practiced sitting and led sedentary lives, Thakuma and Mary remained active at home and work, leading to big rewards in their lives and the lives of their families; true #healthheroes, indeed.

So now we understand that the #healthhero movement results in improved physical and mental wellness. We can increase our longevity and quality of life. What do we do now? It seems that everywhere we turn, there are television commercials, billboards, and Instagram ads about what fitness truly is. Sculpted bodies with chiseled faces seem to be omnipresent. One would think that everyone who is fit is a Greek god or goddess! Is that what a #healthhero should aim for?

Not really. Let's recall that the ideal figure in the not-too-distant past would be considered fat and undesirable today. In fact, what is considered fit and attractive varies throughout the world and is always changing. Beauty is transient and subjective, truly in the eye of the beholder! Our true #healthhero moves with purpose to achieve health and wellness, not to conform to the temporary standards of society.

I include forms of extreme exercise in with these unhealthy trends. The ultramarathon runners and the avid CrossFit practitioner may be healthy and fit, but these regimens are not for all of our #healthheroes. Many of these extreme exercises can lead to injury, as happened with Robert, who suffered a nearly life-threatening complication. Also, they are often not sustainable. It's really difficult keeping up with these fads on a daily or weekly basis. What's critical is that you do what fits in with your lifestyle and goals.

Even though we are inundated with images and information, we must resist and again go back to our purpose. What are we trying to achieve? Are we attempting to be the best parent, physician, teacher, or musician? Once we have this idea firmly in place, we can proceed with confidence to find the movement necessary to attain our goals. In addition, we must shy away from the supplements, diet pills, and fat-burning drinks advertised on every television, Internet pop-up, and bus. Energy is renewed by movement and the metabolism is stimulated to burn faster and brighter.

Fast-track fat-burning methods are advertised on all media fronts. We are bombarded with promises of a quick change from the body we don't want to the "desirable" body we all are looking for! These supplements are often unsafe and unproven. Even the more traditional use of nicotine and caffeine for weight loss is not worth considering by the #healthhero. Smoking two packs of cigarettes daily and drinking coffee all day to maintain your waist size is not sustainable or healthy. The many health hazards cigarettes pose are well known. Maintaining your weight will not take away these risks!

What is healthy for you and something you can do every day? You have to search within yourself and find what fits in your life. Explore. Try different ideas. Also, find something that can be done with a friend or family member. Together, you and your #tribe can motivate yourselves and make your activity more enjoyable.

As a college student in Columbus, Ohio, I discovered group exercise, group movement that a #healthhero often craves. It was the fall of my second year at Ohio State University and I was doing well academically, but wanted to do something that would help my physical and mental fitness. At that time, I wasn't a big fan of working out alone in the gym. Although this was a good plan for some of my friends, it was not my cup of tea.

A friend told me about the group exercise classes that met every evening at six thirty. I was a bit skeptical, not sure this was going to be a fit for me. I went to the first class with my gym bag, a towel, and no expectations. There were seventy-five people in a gym, and I took a place in the middle. The music started as we began our warm-up. The people next to me were smiling and excited. I was surprised. Most people viewed exercise as a chore, something they "had to do." This group was clearly different! For the next forty-five minutes, I was drenched with sweat but filled with energy and vigor. I was really juiced!

I made two friends that day and couldn't wait for the next session. I'd found my way. The energy of this #tribe was palpable. Movement with purpose, that's what this was. I wanted to increase my well-being, and this activity with my new #tribe helped to get me there. I was benefiting from the physical activity and also from the positive nature of the environment. I felt better, emotionally and physically. I was more prepared for my academic challenges as well. This experience helped cement in my mind the importance of movement with purpose, a foundation of the #healthhero.

Many others had already discovered the benefits of group exercise. Your group holds you accountable, helping you stay on the path to good health. The others miss you when you don't show up for class. The social interaction of your #tribe is tremendous. Meeting new people and catching up with your exercise partners is invigorating. Also, keeping yourself motivated toward your fitness goals is often challenging. It is difficult to remain bored if you have a vibrant group keeping your routines dynamic and exciting. Finally, the fitness instructor can help direct your activities, making them safe, exciting, and unpredictable so you don't become bored by any one routine. As a participant in a group fitness class, you can fulfill your #healthhero goals as I did mine!

In my life, I've been most fulfilled and motivated by doing what I really love. Even when I was critically ill as a young boy, I enjoyed listening to cricket matches. Music has been a great love for me as well. Exercise should be the same. If you can find an activity that you enjoy, you are much more likely to do it on a regular basis. Playing basketball was such an activity for me. Hours would pass and I would be engrossed, not worried about the amount of time I spent playing or the effort expended during that time. I continued to perfect my own version of the shot Michael Jordan made or of Allen Iverson's drive to the basket. I simply loved it.

To be a #healthhero, you too can find an activity that you love dearly. You don't have to be an Olympic athlete or have the quickness, strength, or grace of your heroes. You simply have to find the desire and heart. Once you find your favorite activity, do it regularly. Planning is key. You have to make it a part of your life, not a hit-or-miss occurrence. Just as was true about discovering your purpose in life, finding the right exercise takes some searching.

You should ask your doctor for advice on what types of exercise would be helpful and even more important, what is safe for you to participate in. Your health, age, and physical condition all play a role in finding the right activity for you. Once you have some choices from your doctor, you're ready to go. Try a variety of activities to see what tickles your fancy! Also, make sure the activity fits your budget and doesn't require expensive equipment and training, along with coaching.

You can also find personal trainers and health coaches to guide you. They can be valuable resources, instructing you in safe weight-lifting and exercise techniques. Remember, you want to be healthy and achieve wellness, not be out of commission. Weekend warriors are, alas, their own worst enemy. Consistency is the key here.

These trainers can give you the pros and cons of the extreme fitness techniques and help you understand how to efficiently achieve your #healthhero goals. In the United States, many insurance plans have preventive health benefits and may reward you for your fitness activity—an added bonus! Insurance companies understand that if you are proactive and move every day, you are more likely to stay healthy and disease free. Hence, you use fewer services and are a "cheaper" customer. As a #healthhero, you want to be proactive, remain healthy for yourself and your family, and save money. Believe me, insurance rates are not going down any time soon.

Remember that every activity counts! Whether you are running three miles a day or gardening, you are improving your health. That is why taking the stairs, biking to work, and scrubbing the floors are all important. Some of the healthiest populations, those in the so-called Blue Zones, live the healthiest of lives without relying on treadmills, ellipticals, or fancy weight machines.

Dan Buettner studied people living in these Blue Zones, longevity hot spots where the life expectancy was among the highest on our planet. Here, Buettner found folks enjoying life and living long healthy lives without joining expensive gyms, running marathons, or lifting weights. Instead, they moved with purpose, gardening and working in their natural environments with less mechanical equipment. It seemed that the residents of these Blue Zones had surroundings that almost forced them to move for everyday life.

We can follow this concept very well. Instead of hiring a gardener, get out your shovel and rake and work in the yard. Put on a sturdy pair of work gloves and clean up the brush instead of letting someone else do the job. Mow the lawn instead of hiring the neighbor's son to do it. We have many opportunities to mirror the activities of the Blue Zones' residents. You have to make the choice to be a #healthhero and take the stairs, not the elevator; walk in the airport instead of standing on the moving walkway. As long as your body tolerates the activity and your doctor gives the okay, do as much as you can. This will lead to wonderful years spent in the company of your family and friends, enjoying yourself. You will literally be able to live life to the fullest until the end of your life: This is a #health-hero goal.

Far too many of us suffer from chronic diseases, making our twilight years difficult. As a #healthhero, make your priority to move with purpose, with energy. Make it a part of every day so you don't even give it another thought.

PUTTING IT INTO ACTION: PHYSICAL ACTIVITY

Combining your everyday movement activities with formal exercise can be a great combination. What exercises can work for you? Movement and physical activity can be broken down into four basic categories. The first involves aerobic exercise, also known as endurance. Then there is strength training, followed by flexibility and balance training.

Aerobic Exercise

With aerobic exercise, you are using your heart and lungs to improve the circulatory system. You can build healthy lungs and a stronger heart through aerobic exercise such as jogging, participating in an aerobics class or sports like basketball and tennis, walking briskly with weights, lifting light weights in rapid succession (Arnold Schwarzenegger invented this move—with heavier weights—because he hated to jog), dancing, and jumping rope. In addition to a stronger heart and lungs, this form of physical activity and movement will strengthen your immune system, improve your muscle strength, and help prevent disease. Hypertension, diabetes, and obesity can be improved as well.

Interval Training. Recently, interval training has been gaining many fans. You merely undertake 20 seconds of a high-intensity aerobic exercise, followed by a 40-second recovery period of less intense exercise or rest, followed by another 20 seconds of intense aerobics. Repeat, working up to 10 minutes of intervals. Raising and lowering your heart rate in this manner will strengthen that muscle and increase your endurance and strength overall.

Running. In running, interval training is referred to as fartlek, a Swedish word meaning "speed play." Fartlek includes periods of fast running interspersed with periods of slower running. If you jog, sprint for 20 seconds and then return to your normal cruising speed. After 40 seconds pass, sprint again. Repeat throughout your jog, thus increasing the strength of your heart and your stamina.

I loved my aerobic exercise routines even when I was a high school student. I would play basketball and would love the sweat and feel of my heart pumping. Because of my rheumatic heart disease, I had testing to ensure that my heart could handle the workout. I controlled my weight effectively and felt mental stability in times of stress. Aerobic exercise has been helpful to me and countless others. Below are listed some aerobic exercises that may be effective for you.

LOWER-IMPACT AEROBIC EXERCISE

+ Swimming, snorkeling, scuba diving

+ Cycling, stationary and transport

+ Elliptical trainer

+ Walking

+ Rowing

+ Dancing

+ Rapid weight lifting with light weights

+ Golf

+ Ping-Pong

HIGHER-IMPACT AEROBIC EXERCISE

+ Running

+ Jumping rope

+ Performing high-impact routines or step aerobics

+ Tennis, racquetball

+ Hiking

+ Basketball, soccer, baseball, football

- Cross-country skiing, snowshoeing, downhill skiing

- Mountain biking

- Boxing and martial arts

EVERYDAY AEROBIC EXERCISES

- Bike to the corner store instead of driving.

- Take the stairs instead of the elevator. Or get off a few floors early and take the stairs the rest of the way.

- Walk around your building for a break during the workday or during lunch.

- Walk the dog.

- Mow the grass, work in the garden, rake.

- Dance with someone or by yourself.

- Shovel snow.

- Clean the house, basement, or garage.

- Wash the car, vacuum the interior.

Strength Training

Strength training is a type of physical exercise specializing in the use of resistance—weight, whether it's a barbell (free), weight machine, a rock, or your own body weight—to induce muscular contraction, which in turn builds strength. As your muscles get stronger, your body works well. There is a decreased chance of injury and arthritis. You don't always need heavy weights to make this happen. Some level of resistance is all it takes. Furthermore, weight lifting is *the* way to strengthen the skeletal system, an important key to not breaking bones as you age. Those with a high risk of osteoporosis especially benefit from light lifting.

With strength training, you must define your goals. I combine the effects of aerobic exercise with strength training during my workouts. I split my exercise routine between the two, building lung power, blood circulation, and muscle. Building muscle is also important because, at rest, muscle mass burns calories twice as fast as resting fat!

Here are some simple strength-training exercises to get you going.

Hand Grip

This simple exercise should help if you have trouble picking things up or holding on to them. It also will help you open that pickle jar more easily! You can even do this exercise while reading or watching TV. Any activity—from tennis to playing the piano—relies on hand strength.

1. Hold a tennis ball or other small rubber or foam ball in one hand.

2. Slowly squeeze the ball as hard as you can and hold it for 3 to 5 seconds.

3. Relax the squeeze slowly.

4. Repeat 10 to 15 times.

5. Repeat 10 to 15 times with the other hand.

6. Repeat 10 to 15 times more with each hand.

Overhead Arm Raise

This exercise will strengthen your shoulders and arms. It should make swimming and other activities such as lifting and carrying children and grandchildren easier.

1. Stand or sit in a sturdy armless chair.

2. Keep your feet flat on the floor, shoulder width apart.

3. Hold weights at your sides at shoulder height, with palms facing forward. Breathe in slowly.

4. Slowly breathe out as you raise both arms up over your head, keeping your elbows slightly bent.

5. Hold the position for 1 second.

6. Breathe in as you slowly lower your arms.

7. Repeat 10 to 15 times.

8. Rest; then repeat 10 to 15 more times.

Back Leg Raise

This exercise strengthens your buttocks and lower back.

1. Stand behind a sturdy chair, holding on for balance. Breathe in slowly.

2. Breathe out and slowly lift one leg straight back behind you without bending your knee or pointing your toes. Try not to lean forward. The leg you are standing on should be slightly bent.

3. Hold this position for a second.

4. Breathe in as you slowly lower your leg.

5. Repeat 10 to 15 times.

6. Repeat 10 to 15 times with the other leg.

7. Repeat 10 to 15 more times with each leg.

Everyday Strength-Training Activities

✦ When you pick up your child, use it as an opportunity to do a squat. Pick up your child by squatting down, pushing your hips out behind you like you're sitting in a chair, and then driving up from your knees and hips.

✦ Whether you are lifting your cat's litter or a container of laundry detergent, try to fire off 10 to 12 bicep curls. Pause. Recover and do it three times.

✦ Do push-ups against the photocopy machine while waiting for documents.

Flexibility Training

Another form of exercise, flexibility training, helps increase the ability of your joints to move freely and loosens your muscles for exercise as well as daily activities. Although it may not help with strength and endurance, it should be a part of your fitness routine. With flexibility exercises, you can prevent discomfort, especially when you're in a confined space. You will move more gracefully and have less stiffness overall. Yoga is a great example of this type of flexibility exercise.

It was a beautiful spring day and I was ready for the world! I'm sure all of you have had these days, when you felt that you could conquer anything. The flowers were starting to bloom and positive vibes filled the air. I came home, ready for a nice evening with my wife. This was couples yoga night and we were both excited about our evening together. Clad in my Lululemon attire, I was ready to tackle the class with vigor! We arrived at the studio to find dozens of couples, all excited to partner with their significant others in this jubilant evening.

As we moved from downward dog to the sun salutation and warrior poses, we were thoroughly invigorated. Kali and I smiled at each other, our clothes drenched in satisfying sweat! Yoga is a great exercise for the body, increasing flexibility. It is also calming and peaceful to the mind. This form of exercise that originated thousands of years ago in my birth country had traveled with me to the suburbs of the United States. Namaste indeed.

YOGA UNLEASHES THE IMMORTALITY ENZYME

Nobel Prize winner Elizabeth Blackburn of the Salk Institute for Biological Studies found that 12 minutes of yoga a day increases telomerase (the enzyme that slows aging) activity by 43 percent. Work your way up to 24 minutes for a double dose of anti-aging.

Yoga is a mind-body practice originating in ancient India, and it is a great example of flexibility exercise. It integrates both physical and mental practices, with a series of poses, breathing exercises, and meditation. It is easy to do and doesn't require any special equipment. Anyone can participate in yoga, with multiple styles and levels of activity. Your stress levels can be reduced as well as your blood pressure, improving your cardiovascular condition. This is a classic example of East meets West where the #healthhero integrates the best practices from Western culture and Eastern culture to create an arsenal that is effective for achieving health and wellness goals.

Here are some easy ways to incorporate yoga into your daily routine.

Office Yoga

Throughout my day, I sneak off and do yoga. Just a little here and there, and then perhaps some more when I go home later. It all counts, and I find yoga to be the best destressor among all the movements.

Yoga Breathing

This can be done at your desk, in the middle of a staff meeting, or on a train, bus, or plane. Sit or stand with your feet firmly planted on the ground. Take a deep breath, feeling the stomach rise. Pull the air up the spine to the top of your head and then exhale it back out through the nostrils, allowing your stomach to drop. Repeat until you feel calmer and more centered. Yoga breathing is important to master, as it is integral to meditation and relaxation.

Standing Forward Fold

If you've been sitting a long time, this is an effective—and not really noticeable—way to stretch it all out. Simply stand up and drop your shoulders. Pretend your waist is a giant hinge and bend forward. If your hands don't touch the floor, just bend your knees until they do. Bend one knee and then the other, stretching your hamstrings. (You should feel a pull on the back of your legs.) Slowly roll up, breathing slowly all the way, straightening one vertebra at a time, your head and neck coming up last. If possible, go for a second or third round.

Seated Forward Fold

This pose puts the head below the heart, creating a sense of calm and relaxation.

Sit straight in a chair, keeping your feet flat on the floor and placing them slightly wider than your hips. Roll your shoulder blades back and down, keeping your arms at your sides. Pull your belly button in toward your spine to engage your abs. Exhale and bend forward from the hips, slowly lowering your hands to the floor (or to your shins). Slowly round your upper back, lowering your chest into the space between your legs and allowing your head and neck to drop and your shoulders to relax and round.

Stay here for 5 breaths. Inhale and slowly roll up, lifting your head and rolling your shoulders back last.

Wrist Release

This is a great pose for anyone who works on a keyboard frequently.

Extend your right arm, palm down. With your left hand, press your right fingertips toward the top of your right arm. Hold for a few seconds, then repeat the exercise with the other arm. Then flex each wrist in the opposite direction by pressing your fingertips toward the inside of your wrist. To fully release any other tension, extend both arms out and give your wrists a good rapid shake side to side, then up and down.

Seated Neck Rolls

Sit in a chair with your feet planted on the floor, hands on your thighs. Gaze at the ceiling. Begin to roll your left ear toward your left shoulder. Hold for 2 to 3 breaths. Gently roll your head forward so your chin rests on your chest. Hold again for 2 to 3 breaths. Rotate your right ear to your right shoulder, stretching and taking yoga breaths. Roll the head back to where you began, looking upward. Take one more deep breath and continue on with your day, more relaxed and alert.

Seated Mountain Pose

Mountain pose reestablishes equilibrium in the body. It also gives your upper body a nice relaxing, invigorating stretch and engages your core. Throughout this pose, focus on your yoga breathing, stomach rising with the inhale and deflating with the exhale. First, pull your stomach in toward your belly button. Stretch your arms straight up toward the ceiling, shoulder width apart, palms facing each other. Tilt your head toward the heavens and take 5 slow, deep breaths. Drop your arms and relax.

Seated Eagle Arms

This is a great stretch to get to the seemingly unreachable area between your shoulder blades.

Begin by sitting up straight in a chair. Roll your shoulder blades back and down, arms relaxed at your sides. Pull your belly button into your spine to engage your abs, and keep your feet flat on the floor, if possible. Extend your arms out in front of you, bent at a 90-degree angle, forearms intertwined and palms pressed together. Raise your arms until you feel a stretch. Hold for 5 breaths. Then place your right arm under your left and press the backs or fronts of your palms together. Hold for 5 breaths. Then drop your chin to your chest and stretch the back of your neck, taking 5 more deep yoga breaths.

Seated Cat and Cow

Cow and cat are a pair of complementary poses. In the cow pose, you arch your back to stretch the front torso and chest. In the cat pose, you round your back to stretch the back of the torso and the shoulders.

Sit straight in a chair, feet flat on the floor. Roll your shoulder blades back and down, arms at your sides. Pull your belly button into your spine to engage your abs. As you inhale, arch your back, looking up toward the ceiling. Lift your chin and allow your arms to relax next to you. As you exhale, round your spine and let your head drop forward. Tuck the chin and allow your shoulders to roll forward.

Repeat five times, moving fluidly from cat to cow with each deep yoga breath.

The Cobra

You'll have to lie on your stomach for this pose, but if you have the room and the floor is clean, it is transformative, one of the great spine stretches of yoga.

Lie facedown on the floor, the palms of your hands on the floor by your shoulders, the tops of your feet resting on the floor. Inhale as you gently lift your head and chest off the floor. Draw your shoulders back and your heart forward. Don't crunch your neck. Take 5 long deep breaths. Exhale as you slowly lower your body and return to business.

Scale Pose

This engages your arms, upper body, and core, revitalizing and energizing you throughout the day. Sit on a firm chair without arms, your feet flat on the floor. Place your hands palms down on either side of you, fingers grasping the edge of the seat, and raise yourself up for 5 breaths. Drop back to the chair for a few more resting breaths and repeat.

Ankle to Knee

This is one of the best hip-opening poses in yoga. It releases the tightness in the hips that comes from sitting for long periods of time.

To perform this stretch, sit straight in your chair, with both feet planted on the ground. Put your left foot on your right knee, letting the left knee drop open. Keeping your back flat, lean forward to increase the stretch. After 5 to 8 breaths, repeat with your right foot on your left knee.

Hero Pose

The foot is one of the most neglected and crucial parts of the human body. Our feet are the foundation of all upright movement, providing us with transportation, body alignment, and balance. Spend a little time stretching them out and you'll move with more ease and confidence.

Kneel on the floor, the tops of your feet flat on the surface. You may want to use a mat or blanket under your knees or behind your thighs as you lean back. Slowly sit back on your heels, gradually putting weight on the tops of your feet and stretching them out. Sit for 5 deep breaths or as long as you can maintain the pose.

Sitting Reed Pose

Sitting on a chair, lace your fingers together and raise your arms directly overhead, belly button pulled back toward the spine to engage the abs. Gently bend toward one side, feeling the stretch in the other, and take 5 deep yoga breaths. Bring your arms back to center, take 2 resting breaths, and then bend to the other side for 5 more breaths. Return to center.

Standing Backbend

This sounds difficult but is not. Stand facing your desk (or a wall, a countertop, or the back of a chair). Put your fingertips on your desk. Tuck your tailbone in and up, and lean your hips into the desk. Press your fingertips down and with each inhale lift your spine upward, creating length for your lower back. Remember to draw your shoulder blades away from your ears. Feel your chest expanding upward and outward. To come out of the pose, use your fingertips for stability and press your hips away from the desk. Repeat 2 to 3 times.

Seated Twist

Sit with your feet and knees together. Take a deep inhale and straighten your spine. As you exhale, turn your body to the right. Place your left hand on your outer right thigh and your right hand behind you. Be sure to drop your shoulder blades away from your ears. Continue twisting until you can go no farther. Stay for three or four breaths, lifting up through your center as you inhale and moving more deeply into the twist as you exhale. Look over your right shoulder and down toward the floor for an added neck stretch. Repeat the whole twist to the left.

Neck Release

Sitting in a chair, raise your right hand and grasp the left top of your head. Keep your back straight and your belly button pulled toward the spine, engaging your core. Gently begin stretching your head toward your right shoulder, breathing throughout. Do not pull on your neck. Hold this pose for several breaths, return your head to center, and repeat on the other side.

Bound Ankle Pose

This is a perfect way to open your hips as you sit on the floor and watch TV.

Sit with your legs straight out in front of you, raising your pelvis on a blanket if your groin or hips are tight. Exhale, bend your knees toward your pelvis, then drop your knees out to the sides and press the soles of your feet together. Pull your heels in as close to your pelvis as possible, keeping the outer edges of the feet on the floor. With your first and second fingers, grasp the big toe of each foot. Hold for 5 deep breaths. Relax legs and repeat.

Seated Two-Legged Front Bend

Again, try this when watching television with your family. This pose releases tension in the back of the legs and, like all yoga, teaches intention, focus, and patience.

Sit with your legs together out straight in front of you; bend your knees as much as needed to make a forward lean possible. Then lean forward, keeping your back straight, until you feel some resistance in the backs of your legs while you are gently holding your calves, ankles, or feet.

With knees either bent or straight, keep your chest long and open as you continue to lean forward, leading with your belly and lower ribs rather than your shoulders. Take several breaths, lowering your torso toward your legs in this manner, relaxing on your exhales. Round over your legs at the end to release your back and neck.

Each time you grab a little yoga in your day, end it by whispering namaste.

———————————

A "child" of yoga, Pilates is also a great system of exercises to stretch and strengthen the body without putting undue stress on the joints. This exercise program can be done on a mat or on the larger Pilates Reformer, which you'll find in most Pilates studios and gyms.

Here are some flexibility exercises that may help you.

For the Shoulders and Upper Arms

This exercise increases flexibility in your shoulders and upper arms and will help make it easier to reach for your seat belt. If you have shoulder problems, talk with your doctor before trying this stretch.

1. Stand with your feet shoulder width apart.

2. Hold one end of a towel in your right hand.

3. Raise and bend your right arm to drape the towel down your back. Keep your right arm in this position and continue holding on to the towel.

4. Reach behind your lower back and grasp the towel with your left hand.

5. To stretch your right shoulder, pull the towel down with your left hand. Stop when you feel a stretch or slight discomfort in your right shoulder.

6. Repeat at least 3 to 5 times.

7. Reverse positions, and repeat at least 3 to 5 times.

For the Calves

Because many people have tight calf muscles, it's important to stretch them.

1. Stand facing a wall slightly farther than arm's length from the wall, feet shoulder width apart.

2. Put your palms flat against the wall at shoulder height and shoulder width apart.

3. Step forward with your right leg and bend your right knee. Keeping both feet flat on the floor, bend your left knee slightly until you feel a stretch in your left calf muscle. It shouldn't feel uncomfortable. If you don't feel a stretch, bend your right knee until you do.

4. Hold position for 10 to 30 seconds, and then return to starting position.

5. Repeat with the left leg.

6. Continue alternating legs for at least 3 to 5 times on each leg.

For the Lower Back

This exercise stretches the muscles of your lower back. If you've had hip or back surgery, talk with your doctor before trying this stretch.

1. Lie on your back with your legs together, knees bent and feet flat on the floor. Try to keep both arms and shoulders flat on the floor throughout the stretch.

2. Keeping knees bent and together, slowly lower both legs to one side as far as you comfortably can.

3. Hold position for 10 to 30 seconds.

4. Bring legs back up slowly and repeat toward the other side.

5. Continue alternating sides for at least 3 to 5 times on each side.

Here are some daily flexibility exercises that you may find useful:

✦ When watching TV, stretch instead of lying on the sofa.

✦ Do neck and shoulder rolls when washing dishes.

✦ Stretch your quadriceps while standing at your desk.

✦ Stretch your calves when brushing your teeth.

Learn Balance, in Body and Life

Lastly, balance exercises can help the #healthhero maintain stability. They can help prevent falls, a big problem for older #healthheroes. These exercises can help at any age, giving you balance, stability, and confidence in all your activities. Really, any movement that involves staying on your feet helps your balance, and you need great balance for any exercise done upright. Activities that help balance can complement all other types of exercise. Get the body balancing and you will be infused with calm and well-being. Balancing promotes mental focus.

A favorite balance exercise of mine is tai chi. An ancient Chinese discipline, it's a great activity for the #healthhero. It is referred to as meditation in motion! In tai chi, we employ low-impact movements, along with deep breathing; tai chi requires no special equipment or setting and can be done by anyone. It helps decrease stress and blood pressure and increases agility and energy. Thought to unlock the chi, the energy force throughout the body, and balance yin and yang, tai chi is amazing stuff that all of us could use every day in our quest to be a #healthhero.

Incorporating disciplines from across the world to build up the best combination of tools is a must for the modern #healthhero. The quest for wellness knows no boundaries. Load fitness apps on your smartphone to learn new exercises (most apps cost between two and four dollars), watch YouTube videos of movement and exercise, or use a guided workout in which an instructor takes you through the moves on video. Great ideas are everywhere and the #healthhero should never get bored of his or her movement practices. There are just too many fun options available to us today.

Here are more balance exercises for you and your family.

Stand on One Foot

You can do this exercise while waiting for the bus or standing in line at the grocery store. For an added challenge, you can modify the exercise to improve your balance.

1. Stand on one foot behind a sturdy chair, holding on for balance.

2. Hold this position for up to 10 seconds.

3. Repeat 10 to 15 times.

4. Repeat 10 to 15 times with other leg.

5. Repeat 10 to 15 more times with each leg.

Balance Walk

Good balance helps you walk safely and avoid tripping and falling over objects in your way.

1. Raise your arms to your sides, shoulder height.

2. Choose a spot ahead of you and focus on it to keep you steady as you walk.

3. Walk in a straight line with one foot in front of the other.

4. As you walk, lift your back leg. Pause for 1 second before stepping forward.

5. Repeat for 20 steps, alternating legs.

Heel-to-Toe Walk

Having good balance is important for many everyday activities, such as going up and down stairs.

1. Position the heel of one foot just in front of the toes of the other foot. Your heel and toes should touch or almost touch.

2. Choose a spot ahead of you and focus on it to keep you steady as you walk.

3. Take a step. Put your heel just in front of the toe of your other foot.

4. Repeat for 20 steps.

Everyday Balance-Training Activities

✦ Stand up while talking on the telephone.

✦ Stretch to reach items in high places and squat or bend to look at items at floor level.

✦ Use a headset while you are speaking on the phone so you can practice balancing exercises while talking.

✦ Work in the garden—rake leaves, prune, dig, and pick up trash.

By better understanding the importance of movement with purpose, the #healthhero can continue in his or her quest for wellness and excellent health. In the next chapter, our #healthheroes understand the importance of a healthy #tribe, and how to include your #tribe in healthy movement.

30 MINUTES IS THE NUMBER

The University of Copenhagen just studied several hundred slightly overweight men who needed to incorporate a movement routine into their day-to-day life for both health and weight management. The study included a broad interdisciplinary group of researchers who study cultural barriers and entrenched habits.

One group undertook 30 minutes of exercise a day, while a second group did an hour.

Surprisingly, the group that moved for an hour a day lost less weight and body mass than the group that moved for only 30 minutes!

Researchers came to the conclusion that the difference was about time. Thirty minutes was manageable, but many in the second group skipped the hour because of the time commitment.

The real winners were those individuals who walked or biked to or from work or errands. When purpose was folded into movement, time was not a factor.

GETTING STARTED

If you have been glued to the couch a little too much or have let your program lapse, get back at it. Here are a few easy steps to get you back into your 30-minute routine:

1. Get a pair of good comfortable supportive shoes, whether for running, tennis, or walking.

2. Find comfortable clothing that does not get in your way as you move.

3. Begin with 20 minutes a day and work up to 30. If 20 minutes seems too much, start at 15 and work up to 30.

4. Find a "fitness" buddy or friend to help motivate you. An exercise class is good because it meets regularly and you will have others to provide support.

5. Buy a pedometer (they can be found online for less than five dollars) and count your steps. If you start out at 5,000 steps, work your way to 10,000 and then 15,000. It's a slow, satisfying process, and every step counts.

6. Every place is rife with movement possibilities. Doing the laundry? How about some arm curls with that full bottle of detergent? If you catch yourself standing next to the kitchen counter, do 10 vertical push-ups.

7. Dance and play.

8. Fitness is moving away from fancy machines and back to good old hand weights. Invest in a light pair of hand weights (2 to 5 pounds) and set them down where you spend the most time. Work your muscles as you watch television. Fitness is getting blessedly low-tech.

9. Whenever possible, walk, don't ride. Using your legs as transportation is one of the most time-effective ways to fit in great exercise.

10. Be inquisitive. Google. Ask your friends and colleagues what activities they like. Step out of your comfort zone a little. Live!

chapter four

THE #HEALTHHERO #TRIBE

In the age of colonialism, the word *tribe* conjured negative images of wrathful "natives" plunging knife and spear into the sleeping invader. But the world has changed. Our cultural identity is a rising source of pride. Our #tribe, here at *Ask Dr. Nandi*, celebrates differences and honors traditions. We believe in the power of the word and deed: #tribe.

#Tribe is family, bonded by blood. #Tribe is colleagues, students and teachers, bonded by purpose and institutions. #Tribe is neighborhood, the "it takes a village to raise a child" of the African proverb. #Tribe is also random, a "family" made of the people you meet along the course of your life's path who make you laugh, think, enjoy, and thrive. There are informational #tribes (think of the hashtag) and #tribes that bring about social change. The Internet is called the digital #tribe. Some Internet #tribes just want forecasts about upcoming trends in hemlines. Other #tribes may be dedicated to cleaning up the Pacific trash vortex, a monumental undertaking to save that great ocean. #Tribes, then, cluster around all kinds of activities and ideas. My patients are part of my #tribe and I am a part of theirs.

To borrow a phrase from a really great book, in the beginning, we needed #tribes to stay alive. The provision of food and shelter was a never-ending struggle. So were other invading tribes. Religious texts from the Bible to the Koran offer extraordinary portraits of the difficulties of people's lives in ancient times. A strong #tribe meant you might not die under another's sword. A strong #tribe meant group foraging, hunting, and ultimately farming. You might not freeze to death, either. The #tribes' children were raised by the group, involving a wide range of supportive adults. Their purpose was survival. The fact they all formulated religious beliefs and began writing them down in texts is a good sign they considered spirituality integral to the survival of the #tribe. (See chapter 5 for a look at how spirituality impacts the #healthhero.) Even then, humans longed for something bigger than themselves to explain life.

Since the first campfires reflected off our ancestors' faces, #tribes have meant life, and they still do. It's just that science couldn't prove it until recently. In January 2016, a group of researchers at the University of North Carolina, Chapel Hill, led by Kathleen Mullan Harris, found *specifically* that those individuals with strong social networks early and late in life lived the longest. The quantity of social bonds in the middle phase of life was less important. Because of the demands and stressors in this middle phase—career and family building—a small number of highly supportive tribe members were best for health.

"The relationship between health and the degree to which people are integrated in large social networks is strongest at the beginning and at the end of life, and not so important in middle adulthood, when the quality, not the quantity, of social relationships matters," Harris said.

The study, first published in the *Proceedings of the National Academy of Sciences,* evaluated three dimensions of social relationships—social integration, social support, and social strain—in adolescents to those in very old age.

Once social relationships were established, the researchers then evaluated each participant based on four major markers of health: blood pressure, waist circumference, body mass index, and circulating levels of C-reactive proteins, which measure internal inflammation. Those with the smallest social networks scored poorly on biologic testing, indicating a predilection for illness and early death.

A subset of this study—the National Longitudinal Study of Adolescent to Adult Health—undertook one of the largest studies in the field ever when it cross-referenced large amounts of data on social relationships, behavior, environment, and biology and how these forces have an impact on well-being and longevity. Again, the power of friendship was potent.

"We studied the interplay between social relationships, behavioral factors, and physiological dysregulation that, over time, lead to chronic diseases of aging—cancer being a prominent example," said Yang Claire Yang, a professor at the University of North Carolina and a member of the Lineberger Comprehensive Cancer Center. "Our analysis makes it clear that doctors, clinicians, and other health workers should redouble their efforts to help the public understand how important strong social bonds are throughout the course of all of our lives."

FRIENDS?!?

Human beings evolved into #tribes and are highly social animals. We crave contact and belonging. Above that need, friends encourage you to take care of yourself and have your best health interests in mind. This also contributes to why a #tribe—or friendships—keep you healthier.

One study tracked women with ovarian cancer. Patients with lots of social activity had lower levels of proteins that cause the cancer to spread aggressively. Chemotherapy was easier to take and more effective. Friends literally added time to the cancer patient's life.

In another, women with breast cancer who were in a support group lived twice as long as those who were not. Friendships increase your chance of surviving and thriving after a heart attack and can even keep you from catching a cold!

"People with social support have fewer cardiovascular problems and immune problems, and lower levels of cortisol—a stress hormone," says Tasha R. Howe, PhD, associate professor of psychology at Humboldt State University. "[We] are social animals, and we have evolved to be in groups," Howe says. "We have always needed others for our survival. It's in our genes."

Friends!

Even animals forge strong friendships, according to animal behaviorist Temple Grandin. Evolution? Preservation? Sure, Grandin says, but some of them just plain like each other. These friendships range across species—remember the baby rhinoceros and the giant land turtle that bonded after the giant tsunami in the Indian Ocean or the polar bear petting the sled dog?—just as ours do.

The animal world also gives us countless examples of #tribe behavior as well, the most germane being the theory of hive mind. Let's take bees. Yes, bees. (We'll talk birds some other time.) Scientists observing the behavior of bee swarms and life in the colony developed a theory about what they call the hive mind. This hive-mind theory can be applied to almost any large group forging a way forward. Observers watched the bees come to a consensus over hive building and thought that was that.

Enter Thomas Seeley, a neurobiologist at Cornell University, who thought there had to be more to it. He identified the macro hive mind of the swarm and the micro hive mind of each bee. He observed a ritual of head butting between the bees as they came to a consensus on where to build the hive. Too far to the left might mean death to their entire world. Too far right might leave them vulnerable as well. The hive continued to "discuss"—remember that head butt—until they agreed. It sounds like a marriage or a family or a country or a #tribe. The hive mind is reminiscent of a democracy.

Your hive mind is always at work in your #tribe. Each of your brains has many pathways for thoughts to travel, which then move into the larger hive. Ideas of movement, joy, celebration, and service wear off on your hive. You each brush against one another, forming and rejecting ideas and coming to consensus. Good habits beget other good habits or the #tribe exerts pressure.

Science has reported time and time again on the enormous health benefits of social ties. Berkman and Syme (1979) proved that people with the fewest social ties were more likely to die than those who were connected to others.[1] Brummett and colleagues (2001) assessed adults with cardiac disease, and those without ties died 2.4 times faster than those with social contacts. Several recent review articles provide consistent and compelling evidence linking a low quantity or quality of social ties with a host of conditions, including development and progression of cardiovascular disease, recurrent myocardial infarction, atherosclerosis, autonomic dysregulation, high blood pressure, cancer and delayed cancer recovery, and slower wound healing (Ertel, Glymour, and Berkman, 2009; Everson-Rose and Lewis, 2005; Robles and Kiecolt-Glaser, 2003; Uchino, 2006).

Loneliness. While it doesn't sneak in the door with a gun, it kills in its way. The #healthhero keeps his or her #tribe close and also reaches out to others, understanding the need for all people to feel welcome. Some might even become permanent #tribe members.

As you move deeper and deeper into your life as a #healthhero, stay attuned to those who might suffer from isolation or loneliness. Your power lies simply in giving your time and the positive impact is huge.

Play games, deliver a hot meal, take a walk, or run errands for house-bound people. Remember, the elderly and children are especially vulnerable to isolation. Reach out.

I was lucky: I was born in Kolkata on a spring day into a room filled with the love and support of family. It continued through my childhood, adolescence, and young adulthood and goes on to this day. I was blessed from my first breath by the strength of my #tribe. That family I had seen in the middle of the street, making dinner and doing their homework, was blessed with #tribe. My wealthy friend Pradeep was not.

Pradeep was blessed with wealth and economic advantage. His family was quite prominent and well known in Bangalore. We would play at his house; it had a courtyard that was a dream for a little boy. Cricket was more fun there. Soccer teams were easily assembled, with all the kids happily agreeing to come into this little palace. We could find any new toy at Pradeep's first! From the outside, he was living the dream.

However, this was deceptive. Pradeep's father was a successful businessman and left early and came late, never taking the time to even put him to bed. His mother also had a clothing business, not giving her any time to spare. Pradeep was cared for by hired staff, who were polite and made sure he was fed, had clean clothes, and a tidy house to roam about in every day.

A #tribe, however, is about far more than just making sure the basics are met. In Pradeep's case, he had a great deal more than the basics. But Pradeep yearned for the love of his parents and a sense he belonged and was important in their lives. He needed their time to feel that he was a priority, as much as the next building project or clothing design. He was often sad, asking the hired help when his mom would come home or when his dad would be back in town. Love was what he needed to thrive. Don't get me wrong. He had a nice life replete with all the materialistic things, but his spiritual needs were not being met, not by a long shot.

Pradeep struggled a bit in school. He was enrolled in a private school that was demanding even at the elementary school level. He was a bright boy, spewing out the most detailed cricket data on demand! He often daydreamed in class and was in trouble with the teachers and the principal. School administration was less than understanding about the plight of this "privileged" child. Little did the administrator know that the child was far from privileged; he was starved for affection, support, and guidance. #Tribe was missing in Pradeep's young life, a real #tribe, and it was apparent. We need our family and our community to succeed and thrive. So what does a real #tribe do for an individual?

+ #Tribes reinforce your purpose and your sense of belonging, two main themes in your health.

+ #Tribes boost self-esteem and diminish stress.

+ #Tribes improve your sense of self-worth.

+ #Tribes help you deal with trauma, such as the death of a loved one or a divorce in the family.

+ #Tribes encourage you to live in a healthy, positive way, putting on pressure if your drinking escalates or the potato chips never leave your hand.

When I look back at the time I was so sick, I am amazed by the resolve and strength of my #tribe. I also know that if I had been born in the bed next to me—say, Pradeep's—I would not have had this extraordinary #tribe to help pull me back into the land of health. I might have had only maids and butlers by my bedside! So what did they do for me beyond the meals and bedside vigils?

FIRST, UNEQUIVOCAL SUPPORT

And that means not just financial support, but spiritual and emotional support as well. From my days of illness to my hospitalization, I was always propped up by my #tribe. I didn't have to go anywhere to get the help I desperately needed. With this support, I could face the challenges present at every turn. Without this support, I would most certainly have failed to thrive.

There were days when I asked myself, "Why me? Why do I have to be the one stuck at home, not able to go and play or go to school?" My mom and dad always cheered me on, told me how special I was, and made the days at home fun for me. My sister played with me at home, compensating for all those lost days at the playground. My father helped me with my homework, always asking me if I had any difficulties. With this outpouring of love and support, my #tribe helped me to deal with a difficult time that could have engulfed me; instead they helped me rise and become even better from the experience!

SECOND, UNCONDITIONAL LOVE

Throughout my life, my family's LOVE has been unconditional. When I was ill, this was critical. At my lowest point, I was quite depressed. My mom, dad, and sister showed their unequivocal love with their dedication, from my dad's staying in the hospital with me to my mom's making me the best meals so I could have the nourishment needed. I understood that no matter what was happening, what I said, how I felt, or what I did, I was loved.

Along with their kind actions, my #tribe and family spoke to me with words that filled my heart and soul. Even though I knew that I was loved, those words of affection were tremendously important, as they reinforced my perceptions. I'm sure that Pradeep's family loved him, but because they did not tell him so or offer him words of encouragement and support, he had no way of finding this out.

Remember, love changes you chemically. Love releases dopamine, the brain's pleasure chemical, and creates goal-oriented behavior where no one else matters but you and your partner. Touch those you care about or be touched by them, and your body releases the feel-good hormone oxytocin through this dopamine system. Oxytocin calms and bonds a couple together. That jolt of pleasure also reduces blood pressure, speeds healing, and increases pain tolerance.

THIRD, QUALITY TIME

When I fell ill, my dad told his work that he was not going to be available for them until I was well. His priority was me, not the work he loved. Although he was passionate about his work, my father, the brilliant polymer scientist with thirty PhD students, chose to put me first. Obviously, at this urgent time when I had a life-threatening disease, it was essential for my dad to be at my side.

Moreover, whenever there was an important event throughout my childhood and adolescent life, my family was always present. Whether it was a speech given at my school or a competition, my parents could be found smiling in the audience. When I had dinner, my family always sat with me, asking me about what was happening in my life. I always knew that my #tribe would give me the time that I needed whenever I needed it.

FOURTH, TRUE PARTNERSHIP

Whenever I had a new idea or project, I could count on my family for honest opinions and great advice. This included my days as a student and continues today. My wife is an amazing partner in all my life activities, whether they involve our children or our television show. When I was young and we moved to the United States, my father partnered with me to help me thrive in this new culture.

I provide this partnership to my family, including my children and now my parents. The gifts that have been given to me are now being returned to my #tribe. We are closer and our commitment to one another grows each day. My children now appreciate my partnership with them in school, sports, or social activities. They help me test new foods and recipes, serving as a perfect test kitchen team for the growing number of recipes we use to teach nutrition and good eating habits. My kids participate in community events with my wife and me, and I hope they feel a sense of belonging. I help my wife with her life activities as well, giving input and support as much as needed. She in turn has helped me fulfill my dream of providing people with good health information that promotes joy and longer, more fulfilling lives. The exchange of energy and support is always flowing outward and being replenished.

Although a #tribe can do more, the four characteristics above are important for an effective #tribe. You must be willing to involve your #tribe in all aspects of your life. In order to give the benefits and reap them as well, you have to be open to your #tribe's advice and input. The rewards will be phenomenal.

The story of Roseto, Pennsylvania, is a great example of the rewards of a #tribe. In the 1960s, this Italian immigrant village worked together, chatted together on the main street. They would enjoy one another's company and break bread together in traditional Italian meals. Women would work in kitchens making the meals for their #tribe. They supported one another in their #tribes in the face of unsupportive English and Welsh neighbors. The community thrived. In fact, their rates of heart disease were half that of the remainder of the country!

This improved cardiovascular health was independent of their genetics, medical care, or specific medicines. It was the effect of the #tribe on this community. The communal love, friendship, and support were critical to their collective success. The benefits to the community could be objectively measured.

This should come as no surprise. Throughout our history, humans have only survived due to their #tribes and their communities. In ancient times, we worked together for our very survival, but this has changed over time. Our independence has led to separation from our #tribes, who had been essential to our success for over thousands of years. With technology, improvement in transportation, and abundant food and resources, we do not need our #tribes for physical survival. However, without a #tribe, emotional and mental health suffers and can lead to increased disease rates. I am a scientist and a doctor who has felt, more than once, the desire to diagnose a patient as suffering from loneliness, isolation, and a broken heart. As a scientist and a doctor, I wanted to write out a prescription for "more friends."

Dr. Lester Breslow conducted one of the very first studies to link heart disease and mortality with an individual's social systems. Begun in 1964 and now called the Alameda County Study, it was performed in Alameda County, California, and looked for the relationship between social bonds and death rates in 6,928 participants over twenty years.

Those without consistent social contact had almost three times the mortality rate than those with good social relationships.

These results are remarkable, showing the importance of the relationship of the #tribe. Researchers also noted that strong social ties often correlated with a lower instance of the risky behaviors that affect health. Those behaviors were identified as drinking excessive amounts of alcohol, smoking, being obese, sleeping much more or much less than seven to eight hours a night, being physically inactive, eating between meals, and not eating breakfast.

My wife's uncle Rick was a strapping man, full of life and energy. He ran in a community marathon every year. He was forty-two and had a successful business and a family of six, his wife and five children. Rick's world collapsed one day when he was diagnosed with a possibly lethal cancer: sarcoma. Cancer was a word that Rick had never considered having to hear. He had always lived life to the fullest, in both his personal and his professional life.

With his life hanging in the balance, Rick and his family circled the wagons. They decided that Rick would go to the best facility, possibly the best on the planet, to fight this disease and fight hard. MD Anderson Cancer Center was the destination. However, Rick and his family lived in Michigan, and MD Anderson is in Houston, Texas. The family had five children, ranging from nine to seventeen years of age, all in need of their #tribe.

Rick's family was strong, and the #tribe extended beyond the immediate family of six. Karen, Rick's wife, insisted on being with her beloved husband as he headed for the fight of his life. While the fighter headed for the battle with his bride by his side, his family and #tribe held strong. Each of the children was cared for by other family members. Kali's home opened up to Rick's eldest daughter, and she thrived. The other kids also thrived in the arms of their families, in the arms of the #tribe.

In Texas, Rick and his wife fought hard and were successful in beating the cancer. It was no match for his fighting spirit, and he emerged bruised but victorious. His support from his #tribe was critical in ensuring his success. He had someone to talk to, to bounce ideas off of, to take care of scheduling and his day-to-day life. The unconditional love and unwavering support of his wife were essential for his treatment to be successful.

While he was battling for his life, Rick knew that his children were cared for and doing well. He could concentrate on treatments, rest, and healing. In turn, his children were being fed a steady diet of what children need—nutritious foods, structure, and love—and had more to give back to their ailing dad. Without his #tribe, he might not have been able to travel to the premier cancer center in Texas. The partnership of his brothers, sisters, and parents led to his success, so he could thrive. The circle of grace and strength the #tribe provides is forever expanding and replenishing itself. Namaste indeed!

Rick's #tribe was his rock and his support. But what if you don't have this same situation? What if you were not raised in a supportive environment? Are you just out of luck? Not at all. You can create your own #tribe to support, enrich, and love you, and you, them. It requires some soul-searching to find your purpose, as we described previously. Once you have determined what is important, then you are on your way to creating your own #tribe, and in so doing, you are extending your life, your health, and your happiness.

First, what are you looking for? Not everyone is looking for the same things in life. Are you a student trying to find a group to hang with, to have fun and enjoy one another's company? Are you a parent looking for a #tribe that enjoys playing with their children, doing yoga, and having coffee? Are you a senior suffering from joint pain and looking for a support group that values movement and health, loves playing with their grandchildren, and traveling?

Just as important, what do you want to give to your #tribe? What do you have to offer? What are your strengths, and even more important, what are your weaknesses? Are you prepared to be vulnerable and expose your scars? Vulnerability is an enormously important trait for a #tribe, and you should be willing to be vulnerable with them. A #tribe is always about reciprocity: You bring your strengths to them and they to you. It becomes an unspoken fact.

If you're looking for a potential life partner, I suggest you think about him or her as a #tribe leader, a person who shares your values and goals. If you've been with a partner for a long time and want to try the way of the #healthhero, get them on board if you can. Your power—and the great health effects—will grow exponentially.

I found my life partner one fine summer day. Although I'd had multiple conversations with Kali over our dinners, lunches, and trips, I wanted to understand if she would be a part of my #tribe. I thought about our dinner plans and wondered how I would approach the evening. What should I ask? Should I let her know about my dreams? Should I let her know my insecurities and my fears? Looking back now, I smile because I was nervous. Letting someone know your fears and your dreams is a big decision. Like many of you, I'd been disappointed by many others before I met my partner, my #tribe leader. It seemed like Kali would be different, but I could only find one way to discover this. I had to go there and find out.

I spent quite a bit of time looking for the right clothes to wear. I wanted to make sure everything was just right. I wasn't asking for her hand in marriage that evening, but it felt even more important in certain respects. Full of nervous excitement, I drove to the sushi restaurant we were meeting at. It was still light outside as I walked in. I was early and sat down in the far booth. It was unusual for me to be early! Kali would definitely be surprised. I'm a planner when it comes to important meetings, and this was as important as they get.

I always have three messages I want to convey in any meeting no matter how the conversation goes. I learned this from Rhodes Scholar Mike Lanese during my time at Ohio State University. Mike was a tremendous receiver for the football team and was an academic All-American. His words of advice to me would help me for a lifetime. I had my messages written down for my dinner date with my future bride.

Kali arrived and appeared beautiful. I always love watching her enter the room, with perfect grace and dignity. She sat down, and I greeted her with an embrace. After we ordered our drinks, I started a conversation, letting her know that I was thinking about my future and explaining what I felt was important in my life. I was watching her reaction, exceedingly interested in what she would say and do.

I told her that I wanted to leave a bigger footprint on the planet, that I wanted to help change lives for the better. Because this would entail sacrifices for the family, Kali needed to understand this information. Whether it would be through politics or some other form of advocacy, I was committed to making change. Kali smiled and agreed. We should be of service to others in our lives, she concurred.

Babuni, my original #healthhero, had been afflicted with a stroke recently and I wanted to make sure that Kali knew how dedicated I was to my biological family, how I was determined to assist them with my father. Again, this would mean more sacrifice for us, as I spent the nights with my father to help him heal from his illness and thrive again. I did this for six months straight. For a couple just starting out, this could be a significant barrier. My future wife didn't balk at all. She admired my dedication and pledged her support in caring for my ill father. In that moment, I knew that I had found the one, my future and forever #tribe leader.

Not knowing what her reaction would be, I continued to persist in my quest for my life partner, my #tribe leader. Like me, you have to make it known that you are looking for a #tribe. This intention has to be known by others so that you develop your dream #tribe. I don't mean that you should tell everyone you encounter, but rather the folks that you feel are special, those that you feel are real candidates.

Start with your biological family. Although your biological family should be a part of your #tribe, this doesn't always happen. As was true of Pradeep, your biological family may not be your true support system. If you find that your family is not your rock, then make the effort to change that. Find commonalities among family members, things that bind you besides biology. Let them know what you feel is important and real, and ask them what they find to be of critical importance in their lives.

Then find some fun stuff that you can do together. Get to know your parents and your siblings so you can really have fun together. If your brother enjoys sports, take in a baseball game and enjoy each other's company. The time you take to understand each other will be quite amazing, and your relationship will blossom. With any luck, he will attempt to do the same with you.

Because you also share a common biology, the bonds will only be stronger. Many families have never spent the time to do this and suffer the consequences. The "bed you were born into" may be difficult, but your original #tribe—your family of origin—will always hold a key piece of your identity, positive or negative. To engage with them, find points of common interest and perhaps serve as their #healthhero. The higher you rise in your commitment to the #tribe, the higher the world rises in compassion and empathy.

Just because you share blood ties doesn't always mean your blood relatives are your best #tribe members. Make sure that those you choose to be in your #tribe lift you higher and you do the same for them. Your cousin, the one so critical of your goals, may not be the best support person to have in your life. Once you determine your life's purpose, then you can decide which people you want close to you. You have to be honest with yourself and those around you. The people that you've spent so many years of your life with may not be the best people for your #tribe.

Joining a healthy #tribe is also very important. You may find a group that is fun-loving and spend time having a good time, but this #tribe may not be healthy for you. (Remember the Alameda County Study from earlier in the chapter?) You must ask yourself, "Am I being supported by them and pursuing my goals? Am I supporting them and their goals?" Many groups foster unhealthy behaviors of the mind and body, ultimately not being the #tribe of the #healthhero.

Like life, the #tribe grows and ages and the young take on leadership roles. That's what happened when my #tribe stepped in and saved me!

––––––––––––––

The dawn began to break in northern Michigan and the lake slowly awoke from its warm night of rest. Birds were chirping and the fishermen were planning a trip. In our cottage, we were all starting our day. My nieces were preparing to go fish with their grandpa, their hearts and minds filled with hope and their faces filled with smiles.

I awoke to the words "He's not breathing!" I leaped up, ready to assist. The words brought back the years of residency training at the Detroit Medical Center, where I covered night call every three nights for month after month. I would be awakened by the loud and caustic sound of the beeper and the voice of the nurse: "He's short of breath," or "She's having chest pain."

Back in the days of my residency, I would jump out of bed and hurry to the floor to evaluate the emergency. It became instinct, and I was ready to act on the patient's behalf, as his or her advocate, as his or her #healthhero. Those nights shaped me to become the physician I am today! So it was not surprising to see me jump right up, ready to assist the patient who needed my help.

"Who is not breathing?" I asked.

"You are not breathing!" my family exclaimed.

"What?! There must be some mistake!" I told them.

"No," they all confirmed. "You were not breathing at all for a LONG time."

Wow, I thought. *Could I have a serious problem?*

I was aware that I snored, but this was the first I had ever heard about not breathing. Could I have a sleeping disorder? For the past several months I had felt fatigued, but I attributed that to working hard. I was more tired in the afternoon, but I powered through just fine. As a child I had watched my dad not breathe for a couple of seconds at a time after he fell asleep; he also snored.

Upon returning to our home in metro Detroit, I wanted to find the reason for this surprising cessation of breathing. I started my testing with a sleep study. This involved my going to a sleep lab, where I was connected to wires and devices to measure my breathing, my heart rate, and the oxygen levels in my blood. "There's no way I'm falling asleep with all this stuff on me," I said sarcastically to the technician. I called my family and sent them pictures of me with all the devices connected.

The next thing that I remember was waking up to my alarm. It was six thirty the next day. I guess I'd been wrong. After getting dressed, I asked the technician how I did on the sleep test. "I can't give you any results," she said with a smile, "but try not to sleep on your back." "Okay, great," I said. "I must have a sleep disorder." That was not what I wanted to hear.

A couple of weeks later, I visited the office of the sleep doctor to go over the results of my eventful sleep study. He greeted me with a nice handshake and a warm smile. "Please have a seat, Partha," he said. I sat on the comfortable chair and listened. "You have obstructive sleep apnea," he told me, "and it's not mild." *That's just great,* I thought. I found that I stopped breathing or became apneic several hundred times a night! My oxygen saturation went down to the low 70s percentage, with the high 90s being normal. "So, Doc, my body wasn't getting the oxygen it needed, was it?" I asked. He nodded in agreement.

It all made sense now. The afternoons when I became tired and had difficulty with fatigue were all a consequence of this disorder. The doctor became the patient! Again, I was on the other side of the table, forced to understand the plight of the patient. I was going to be a #healthhero and attack this problem. Soon I returned to the sleep lab, this time to get treated for my sleep apnea.

"I'm back." I smiled as I greeted the technician.

"I kinda thought you would be," she said with a half-smile.

This time I was fitted with a device that went on my nose to help me overcome my difficulty. The technician made some adjustments and gave me a setting. The nasal prongs, a bit like the oxygen cannula given in the hospital to patients, were even bigger. *This is gonna be fun,* I thought. I was going to do it! Closing my eyes tightly, I tried to fall asleep.

I sat up bolt upright, sweating from a bit of panic. The nasal prongs had given me a feeling of claustrophobia, and I experienced anxiety. I began to have feelings of doubt creeping in. Could I do this? Then I closed my eyes and had a quiet moment of meditation. I began to center myself and visualized the situation. *This is not difficult,* I thought. *I want to be alive for my kids' graduations, their weddings.* With my sleep apnea, I was at risk for heart attack, stroke, high blood pressure, and irregular heart rhythm! This #healthhero had to survive.

I put the nasal prongs back on and took some deep breaths. I thought about my #tribe and my training to be an advocate and champion. I had taught them and they me. After all, I wouldn't have known I had quit breathing if my #tribe hadn't been there, aware and focused! The students were now the teachers, the wonderful circular nature of the #healthhero, always learning and giving back. The next thing I remember was the morning alarm. Invigorated with my victory, I was ready to get to work and attack the day. My practice and experience had paid off!

In the coming months, I understood firsthand what it meant to be reenergized. The vital importance of sleep became obvious to me. Sleep is important for repair and rejuvenation, I had learned in medical school and residency training. Sleep is brain food, really. The #health-hero's brain functions optimally with quality sleep. The rest of the body also performs much better with the right amount of sleep. Blood pressure is more regular, and individuals who have adequate amounts of sleep are less likely to be obese. Even the immune system functions better with the right amount of sleep. I noticed that my moods were stabler, as was my emotional balance. The doctor as the patient, a #healthhero patient, was quite an interesting experience indeed.

———————

The spring evening air was cold and we were ready to call it a night. My sister was discussing the merits of the Democratic candidates for president, Hillary Clinton and Barack Obama. We were deep in the throes of discussion when my dad came and told us, "Don't waste your energy and breath. They're both politicians." My sister and I looked at each other and agreed. Babuni was right. Little did we know that he would never have that level of clarity of thought and speech again.

Shortly after this time, we went to my father's room, startled by sounds that we heard. Upon entering, I saw my dad struggling to speak, his speech slurred and his face drooping. "He's having a stroke," I cried, and asked my family to find aspirin. My father was my #healthhero, the man who had stayed with me in my time of greatest need. I never questioned what I would do for him; he was my #healthhero and I would be his. Our purpose was constantly shifting based on who needed help to get well.

He went to the hospital, and our fears were confirmed as we learned the damage the stroke had done. Through the months and years, my sister, mother, and I learned to be health advocates for my father. We were his #healthheroes, fighting to give him the best treatment despite the insensitive words of the insurance companies, who wanted to stop care. We fought against apathetic caregivers and insisted they perform.

The cultivation of our minds helped us to overcome our challenges in caring for our dear father. The spirituality of our #tribe was strong. We prayed and meditated as we supported and nurtured the patriarch of the family, showering him with love and compassion. The #healthheroes of our #tribe found their inner strength through our combined spirituality and support.

One of our challenges in caring for our father was the lack of support we found in the health-care system. I had a lot of difficulty with the lack of compassion. My father's severe stroke led many to write him off and declare him unfit for life on this planet. My dad was not alone. Countless folks in our nation and around our planet suffer due to lack of adequate care and compassion. The #healthheroes' efforts at advocacy for themselves and their loved ones is critically important. A simple urinary tract infection not treated properly can lead to disaster. An incompatible group of medications can lead to life-threatening complications.

The #healthhero steps into this gap, providing the time and care that all human beings need, deserve, and should receive. The sick should get whole healing foods. They should not be alone. They should be wanted and loved. Medical institutions don't provide support and kindness, so we must provide them, as much as we can, to keep healthy, focused, attached to other people, and full of purpose.

PARTHA'S RX

1. #Healthheroes with a great #tribe can achieve improved health. In fact, your #tribe can improve your heart health and immune system!

2. A #healthhero finds a #tribe that has healthy behavior. Your #tribe will reinforce and support this behavior, increasing well-being for you and your #tribe.

3. #Healthheroes may have different #tribes in different phases of their lives. Find the #tribe that helps support you through your challenges and victories.

4. Remember, the best #tribe of the #healthhero may not be his or her biological family. Understand who you are and what you need and can give in a #tribe in order to select the #tribe that is right for you.

So the #healthhero must create a core group of people that forms his or her inner circle, a true #tribe. This may contain your blood relatives, as is true with my family, but may also include others, principally your life partner. Choosing a life partner is really choosing the leader of your #healthhero #tribe. If you haven't found your life partner, that's okay. Identify the strongest parts of your #tribe, the individuals who share traits and habits that you find to be critical in your life. You may find your special #healthhero and #tribe member at work or on your softball team or in your painting class. Be open to realizing that the possibility of life enhancement exists with these relationships. Be open to the idea that each new person you meet may be a future key member of your #tribe. Or not. That's part of the beauty and mystery of life.

Residents of Okinawa, Japan, are known throughout the world for their longevity. People regularly live into their nineties and hundreds. Along with a great diet, they have a wonderful support system in which groups really look out for one another. They have a marvelous tradition called *moai*. Moai is a group created by people to offer emotional, social, and financial support to one another. It developed when farmers had meetings designed to help each other understand how to grow the crops with the best yield and efficiency and also how to deal with the times when crops did not grow.

Presently, the people in a moai are in an extended family of sorts. They plan together and combine their talents and resources. When one member is down on their luck, others step up and take up the slack. When you belong to a moai, you feel as if you're not alone, that your people will be there for you, in good times and bad. This feeling of belonging is important and can be vital.

Members of a moai live longer and live well! This is great news for the #healthhero! Folks belonging to a moai have behaviors that foster good health. Healthy behavior is contagious.

What do I mean by *contagious* here? If a member of your #tribe has amazing healthy habits of diet and exercise, this is passed on to the others in the group. Quickly, the enriching behavior is the standard by which the entire #tribe lives every day. Wellness can be pursued and achieved with the help of the moai, the #tribe.

Not only are the members of the moai living physically healthier lives, they are happier as well. Remember that as human beings, we need emotional and social connections for our health and happiness—indeed, for our overall well-being. The social support that these moais or #tribes provide is crucial for the #healthhero.

Stress is also not much of a concern for the Okinawans belonging to their moai. Like all of us, these members of the moai have stresses that affect their lives. Unlike many of us, their #tribe members are very involved, spreading the increased stress over several people. Whether it's an unexpected tragedy due to death or disability or a child-rearing issue, the members of the moai jump in to help, relieving the added burdens. This decreased stress helps their health, both physically and emotionally, another must for the #healthhero. Remember, stress causes inflammation, and inflammation causes disease.

Like our global Okinawan neighbors, we need our moai, our #tribe. It will take time to build a great one for yourself. But you can't sit idly by waiting for something to happen. In today's very connected world, finding a #tribe may be easier than ever. It can also be deceptive. Social media can be quite superficial and serve as bragging sites for some.

Beauty secrets and clothing posts can be entertaining but don't provide cultural enrichment. I feel that social and digital media can be deeper if you choose it to be so. Just as you are selective with your real-life friends, you can be just as discerning with your social media pals. Your posts, tweets, and snaps can be specific or broad. With time, you can attract different peeps with your goals and heart. Connecting can be meaningful whether it is to someone down the street or a friend thousands of miles away. Engaging with a #tribe that has your back is a wonderful tool in creating a successful, long, joy-filled life.

The Royal Society (beroyal.com) is an online community, a #tribe where members are supportive, nurturing, and loving. In a planet where affirmation of a person's worth is not always given and where individuality is not always fostered, this social media community gives its members the love and support that they often don't find elsewhere. The intent behind the group is to live royally, with members treating one another with respect and admiration. The community leads its members to understand how much they are cherished. This leads to amazing feelings of belonging.

Founded by Bryant McGill and Jenni Young of SimpleReminders .com, the Royal Society has Royal Meet ups, where they travel together to a new location, to discover the place and their Royal comrades. On a cool late summer day, fourteen of the Royals came to Detroit to visit us. We were thrilled to meet them and show them our community, our world, along with the joy that this town brings to us. They were driving and flying from Texas, Ohio, Indiana, Canada, and northern Michigan.

First stop on the Royal Detroit Meet up was in the studio of WXYZ ABC Detroit, where we split up the fourteen into two groups. We showed them how I work and the wonderful magic that happens in a television station. I explained the process of broadcast news to them, while showing them the bright lights of the studio, the grind of the newsroom and "go time," what it's like to be live on television with little room for error.

Next we stopped in downtown Detroit. Long the butt of jokes and ill-timed publicity, coupled with the lack of great leaders, our city had taken a beating in the press. The Royal Meet up thrived in the heart of downtown Detroit. This #tribe took it all in, pleasantly surprised by their surroundings. In the midst of this exploration of the Motor City, we were sharing a wonderful meal, laughing and learning about one another. Our stresses were taking a hiatus and our souls were full. This moai, originating from the online platform created by Mark Zuckerberg, had come to our planet, enriching our lives.

You can create your own #tribe, much as the Royal Society has. You must clearly want to reach like-minded others. Your vulnerability and genuine need to connect should be transparent in your social media. Your posts should let others who are also searching for a #tribe know that you want to support them and be supported. Obviously, you have to be selective but open-minded.

A family friend related a story about her adventures on Twitter that enriched her life. Through sheer happenstance, she had an exchange with a high school student in Benares, the holy city in India where the dead are returned to the Mother Ganges. She expressed a desire to visit the city but doubted she'd ever make it. Raj, her new Twitter friend, activated his fellow students and soon her in-box was filled with pictures of their hometown they had taken over the years, its temples, funeral pyres, and holy men. They explained what was happening in the pictures and what their culture believed. Her heart opened wide through the sheer wonder and miracle of it all. How could she be in America and India simultaneously? Why were these high school students taking the time to show her their world? This new Benares #tribe is about to graduate from high school and she's looking forward to seeing their pictures of Goa, the beach resort where they will take their graduation holiday. Just because she was open-minded, her world expanded and her digital #tribe grew.

#Tribe building is sometimes the result of a happy accident. I was in my first year of practice and had just finished my medical training, ten years of intense training *after* finishing college. Excited about the future, I worked hard, coming to the hospital early and leaving late. On one of my evening rounds, I met Steve, an internist who was also looking to establish his career.

Steve and I saw a lot of each other, sharing our victories and frustrations, laughing about the late-night calls from the hospital. Once I was called at 3:00 a.m. to inform me that a patient had a bowel movement! Steve "got it" and empathized with me. Over time, he became a part of my #tribe. We went to basketball and hockey games and conferences. We shared stories of our families, both biological and work! Our #tribes began to overlap and this broadened our social contacts and made our lives more fun.

When his children were born, I felt as if they were my own. What started as an evening hospital encounter transformed into an introduction to a #tribe member. Just as important, we allowed other individuals to understand the importance of our relationship, our willingness to support each other. As #healthheroes, we aren't rainy-day friends; our relationships are our gold.

It's not necessary to have only one #tribe. Your work #tribe may be different from your home #tribe. Your work family can help you with different goals, sometimes more effectively than your spouse. As happened for me with Steve, you can both understand and lend a helping hand, an attentive ear and words that heal. A #healthhero can form different #tribes to meet different needs in life. In the different phases of your life, your needs change and you must be flexible enough to address these. Even in a single stage of life, a #healthhero must be able to go between different #tribes easily, always keeping your goals and principles in sight as well as those of your other #tribe members.

A core group may emerge in your #tribe, with members from different groups coming together. However, this is not necessary. As long as you maintain your passion and figure out your goals with your partners, that is all that is needed. No rules exist in finding your #tribe or #tribes, other than the rules you set. The universe is full of extraordinary #tribes waiting to be formed by you and with you.

Keep it fun and energizing! That is the theme for our #tribe's activities. Although you and your group support one another with strength and passion, do your best to make your #tribe a fun-loving group. This will keep you together through some of the rough times. By mixing it up, you create a more dynamic #tribe, filled with adventure and spirit.

My wife's grandfather Leon and her grandmother Sally loved Michigan State University. At every basketball game and football game and tailgating opportunity, they were a fun couple, often laughing and celebrating. They shared their love of life with each other. Leon and Sally had a group of couples, their #tribe, who enjoyed many of their fun times with them. Drinks in hand, they laughed and cried together. They watched and celebrated one another's lives, forming a strong bond.

Kali and I were invited to several games and watched them as they expressed their mutual joy and love. Sally, historically the life of the party, had a sparkle even in her older years, looking at me with real warmth and affection. Leon shared stories of Magic Johnson, the legendary basketball player with Michigan State and later the Lakers. "So, Partha," he would say to me, "did I tell you the time that Magic wiped the floor with a towel he took from the bench? They won that game handily after that moment!"

The stories weren't as important as his desire to introduce me to his #tribe. He was reaching out to immerse me in the world that he knew, introducing me to the people he called his friends and his support. It was wonderful and helped me to reach him, to empathize and really know Leon.

Years later, when Sally passed away, the entire #tribe was there to console Leon, to support the family and let them know how special my wife's grandmother truly had been to them. We were deeply saddened by her passing but so appreciative of our memories of her. That is what a family does. Almost all our memories of Leon and Sally are of fun times, laughing at Leon's amazing stories and being charmed by Sally. When Leon became ill with heart disease, we were more than happy to ensure that he received the best care possible. That's what the #tribe of the #healthhero does in times of need.

Like Leon and Sally, Kali and I have a lot of fun. My #tribe leader and I enjoy each other's company. We spend as much time together as possible, despite our busy schedule. We enjoy concerts, from Jay-Z to Coldplay. I love dancing at these concerts, and my graceful bride, who minored in dance, helps make the evening a wonderful experience. Sports events are also a favorite.

I get a little excited at the Lions and Pistons games. After a score, I love high-fiving our neighboring seat holders, and by the end of the game, we have made some new friends! Kali is a great companion at these fun events, with a big smile and an awesome attitude. We work to make these experiences amazing for ourselves. Loads of fun with my life partner! Namaste indeed.

Cooking with my bride is also a blast. We organize our time and shop for ingredients, making a conscious decision to obtain the best foods for our family, our #tribe. As we do this, our bonds grow stronger. In addition, we all eat healthier. Our group behavior helps us all stay with our plan to avoid many temptations. As I discussed earlier, the #tribe's behavior helps all the members. Healthier behavior then results for everyone.

#Tribes evolve and grow with their experiences, thus becoming more effective. Each member brings new ideas and different ways of accomplishing tasks—as, for example, our boys do when they add new twists to the food we make or to our exercise routines. The variety of new experiences keeps the family invigorated, leading to the growth and strengthening of the entire group. New bonds are created, all critical to the #healthhero, and lead to improvement in the physical and mental health of all the #tribe members.

Before I met my wife, I loved to exercise, playing basketball and tennis. Although I wasn't an avid runner, I did enjoy jogging as well. After I met Kali, my #tribe leader, I became more fully acquainted with an ancient form of workout of both mind and body. Originating from my country of birth, yoga is an invigorating form of exercise formulated over centuries to prepare the body for meditation. Today most Western yoga classes have only a short meditation period at the end of class; they need to keep those classrooms filling and refilling. But the practice of yoga is about preparing the body for contemplation; the great workout is a happy bonus.

When we were deep in our courtship, I asked Kali what she would consider her favorite activity. Near the top of her list was yoga. I was intrigued and asked her for more information. She loved how yoga made her feel: invigorated and energized, ready to conquer the world.

She described the strength of body and mind needed for this ancient practice. It brought her peace and stillness in the midst of a chaotic world. So I decided to pursue this experience with her. Here I had never practiced yoga before and I was born in India, the birthplace of yoga! I too wanted this #healthhero tool. In chapter 3, I mentioned the benefits of yoga, many of which are critical to the goals of health, wellness, and longevity. I started to practice at home with some introductory moves. It felt wonderful. She was right, I thought.

So we began practicing together. What a blast! I became closer to my life partner and appreciated a part of her life. I could do this only because I was open and ready to accept change. Accepting my #tribe member's experience, I enhanced my own existence. My mind and body, yearning for new challenges, were satisfied, thanks to my #tribe. The #healthhero continues to proceed toward the goal of health and wellness.

I learned at a young age that becoming stagnant, stuck in your ways, is a recipe for failure. My mom and dad taught me to be resilient and adaptive. We moved from Kolkata, India, to Bangalore, a dramatic change in culture, with different foods, language, and customs. My father and mother took it in stride, adjusting to the culture rapidly.

Soon we were eating sambar and vada, a South Indian favorite. We began speaking Kannada, the local language. Being versatile, while maintaining our roots, was a great lesson for our #tribe. It helped us become stronger, gaining more members for our #tribe as well as expanding our minds and hearts. And because we were so strong a #tribe, we could do it. We could enter a new culture and thrive despite the uncertainties. Although at first this was uncomfortable, these challenges made way for our strength in our family, both biological and extended.

In the midst of these changes, amazing consequences occurred for the #tribe. We were able to support one another even more. The ideas that bind us together become actions and lead to a stronger future. Challenges in parenting, job performance, or academics all become small with the help of your #tribe. The #healthhero prevails, overcoming obstacles with the help, love, and support of his or her #tribe.

As a young #healthhero, at the age of nine, I entered the United States full of expectations and wonder. Unfortunately, I found the adjustment to this new environment to be challenging. Seemingly simple cultural norms were a barrier for me. Kids my age were less than understanding about my lack of cultural knowledge of American norms.

My classmates laughed at my clothes, and because we had never used deodorant in India, I was often ostracized and bullied. Kids were demeaning in their language and I was often alone. I felt alone and somewhat helpless. In this situation, my biological family, who were also adjusting to the culture, found it difficult to help me at first. Although the new nation held such promise and I was filled with wonder at the possibilities, my daily existence at school and play was miserable. I was given the proverbial gut check at a vulnerable age.

I struggled to find some relief from the abusive environment. It seemed like I was waiting for the next biting comment to come, always uncomfortable in all situations. I searched for support and comfort, and a few months into my ordeal, I found some relief. Mike and Robert were good kids and understood my plight. They gave me advice to deal with my difficulties and protected me from some of the bullying. As time passed, we became quite close.

Despite our vastly different backgrounds, we gelled well. Mike was from an affluent African American family and Robert was Caucasian from a poor family. We were a motley crew indeed, but a strong unit nevertheless. We provided support to one another, growing as individuals and as a group. We celebrated together and lamented our losses together. With each adverse event, we seemed to become stronger, our #tribe becoming more resilient.

These boys helped shape the minds and hearts of their #tribe, our #tribe. And this resilience was not unique to our group. Just like the Italian immigrants in Roseto, Pennsylvania, our #tribe became strong when faced with adversity. Studied for decades by scientists, Roseto had lower rates of mortal illness such as cardiovascular disease and heart attack than all the surrounding towns. The reason had nothing to do with health care or drinking water or air quality. The people of Roseto lived longer lives because of their tight communal bonds: They were nourished by other people.

Our young group thrived together. We helped each other and became healthier in our minds and our bodies. We had a bit of swagger and understood the collective power of our group. In Roseto, the previously described immigrant Italian population was an outlier, with remarkably decreased heart attack rates despite dietary indiscretions. My young buddies and I were outliers too, thriving despite our circumstances.

#Tribes can thus be tremendously valuable in the midst of challenging environments. My wife and I always loved the idea of raising children together. As any parent will tell you, raising kids will test—and require—almost all your abilities. Waking in the middle of the night with an infant or toddler is just the beginning. There are the temper tantrums and the seemingly irrational choices your child makes. All of these situations provide a time of reflection and growth for your #tribe.

Kali and I don't always agree on every decision, and we compromise to form our collective opinions. With each disagreement comes growth for our family. Like our growing family, we grow with them, becoming more resilient, more supportive. That is the beauty of a #tribe: Something small takes root and grows big and strong against sun, rain, and wind.

This is especially true due to our diverse backgrounds. Both my wife and I are blessed with supportive parents from different corners of the planet. This blending of cultures, ideas, and strengths is ideal for the twenty-first century. Our world has become smaller, with ideas from multiple cultures becoming incorporated quickly throughout all our societies. With our eclectic group of family members, our #tribe is adeptly equipped to survive and thrive!

Our variety of ideas and thoughts, drawn from ancient cultures as well as modern civilizations, is quite timely for the #healthhero. Faced with a dizzying array of fads and thoughts, the Snapchat generation is always yearning for the next best idea. Understanding the beauty of the #tribe is very important. Like the residents of Roseto, who under the guidance of their #tribal leaders protected their rich traditions of Italy, we too can preserve the beauty of our cultures and our traditions. The #healthhero can achieve his or her goals of improved wellness with such perseverance. While information can be transmitted in a nanosecond, the work of the #tribe is timeless.

My #tribe gathers at Long Lake in Michigan, a remarkable place. It is where we come to be together in nature, building memories and reinforcing our feelings and our bond. There are no bad days here, no stress. The beauty of the lake, located in the northern part of Michigan, is obvious and unchanging. I revel in its blue water and green banks. It still amazes me every time I see it. Kali had spoken about this place, her family's cottage on Long Lake, during our dating days. It's a nice four-hour drive from the suburbs of Detroit, and the journey takes your mind and your body to a different state. Our family visits several times a year, typically in the late spring, summer, and early autumn.

As we approach the cottage on the lake, we slow down. The beauty of the trip is astonishing. Greenery and pristine lakes remind us of our amazing world, a gift of mind-boggling proportions. On turning into the cottage, we are greeted with the sign on the front: A PIECE OF THE ROCK. We all smile when we see this. We have arrived in this beautiful quiet place in which we have done so much bonding.

The kids run out with big smiles. They are excited to see their grandparents, their cousins. Only a few minutes go by before they are asking to jump in the water. Life is simpler here. My father- and mother-in-law have worked diligently to create a world for their #tribe, one that is unfettered, unfazed by the Instagram moments of the day. Like the Roseto families, we are three generations sleeping under one roof, cooking in a communal kitchen.

EIGHT HUGS A DAY FOR A LONG, JOYFUL LIFE

Studies have showed time and time again that hugs keep people healthy, help add years of life to the elderly, and make giver and recipient feel good.

Here's a little we know about the health-giving magic of hugs:

+ Every hug boosts your oxytocin levels and helps heal feelings of isolation, loneliness, and anger.

+ Holding a hug for a longer amount of time releases more serotonin, boosting mood and feelings of happiness.

+ Hugs build trust, boost self-esteem, and relax the nervous system.

+ Well-hugged babies grow into less stressed adults, and we have ample science to understand the horrifying health consequences of prolonged stress.

+ Like meditation and laughter, hugs reconnect you to the moment and teach you to let go, connecting you to health and joy.

We all take turns preparing meals with each generation, making breakfast, lunch, and dinner. The kids help with caring for the littlest ones. Time has stood still, in some respects. Board games hold much promise for a great time. We have a television, but I don't remember watching it. Conversations during the day, about life in general and about our trials and tribulations, are often the highlight of the trips.

Then there is the pristine beauty of the lake. This is what our #tribe loves about our place up north, which is what we call this haven. Our children, the same technology-loving individuals from the urban environment, are in heaven. They are jumping in the water, zipping about on Jet Skis, and enjoying the simple pleasures of life. Their grandparents in their #tribe have created this place to show their love, their support, and their spirit to the family.

The nights are just as much fun. Campfires up north are wonderful. What originated as a way to provide warmth and light has now become a focal point for our nocturnal activities. The kids gather the material needed for the fire as instructed by their grandpa Rocky. The fire is started and then the marshmallows are roasted, much to the children's delight. We finish the marshmallows and the kids go slowly up to the cottage to sleep. They give mild resistance, eager to stay up with the adults.

Then the real campfire conversations begin. We laugh and tell jokes and stories, and general bonding occurs. The #tribe laughs, cries, and connects in this simple environment. We celebrate the beauty of our relationships, with simplicity. The cool trends of the day, the transient fads are not important. Rather, the traditions of a thousand years are paramount—family and friendship, love and support. It's quite beautiful to watch. The #healthhero basks in the beauty of the #tribe.

In fact, we will pass this tradition to our children and hope they will do the same for theirs. Our #tribe will grow stronger with time, building momentum and strength. This legacy of building #tribes is fantastic, and it's what the Okinawans have done for generations. With our simple practices shared by our family, we begin this process and cement the importance of our relationships and support. We encourage and empower the younger members of our #tribe so they can be better every single day. The #healthhero can then pass on his or her habits of #tribal wellness to multiple generations.

With the #tribe firmly in place, the #healthhero is ready to go to the next level. In the next chapter, we will discuss how the #healthhero's spirituality puts him or her on the path to achieve great health and wellness.

PUTTING IT INTO ACTION: HELPING KIDS FORM HEALTHY #TRIBES

As soon as a child smiles at his or her mother or goes on that first playdate, a #tribe is being formed. Family hopefully provides the foundation of a child's #tribe, offering a safe, loving place to learn and grow. Other members will join along the way, from school, sports teams, committees, and schoolyard friendships. Favorite teachers or other adults may join your child's #tribe as well.

As the #healthhero of your #tribe, your job is to know who is in your child's life, how they think and behave. Positive respectful interaction is the key. Talk to your kids. Make it your business to know their friends and their friends' parents. Keep the lines of communication open, and when difficulties arise, use them to teach valuable lessons. Some of your child's #tribe will come and go as they develop. #Tribe building is a key element to long-term health, happiness, and success in all parts of life.

Offer your children as many activities and expose them to as many cultures as possible. Let their passions form their #tribe and their #tribe will stoke their passions.

How Your #Tribe Influences the Course of Your Life

The bed you were born in is just that, the beginning. You may start life with a difficult #tribe who cannot support and enrich you. Sometimes leaving one #tribe for another or building your own is the only way. A negative, unhappy, or unethical #tribe will pull you down and create problems in life. Self-esteem suffers.

A positive, happy, and morally aware #tribe lifts you up and brings out the best in you. Pay attention to the behaviors of your #tribe and how you feel around them. Use your heart and head as your guide. No matter how painful it may seem at the time, remove or distance yourself from #tribe members who do not make you a better you.

PLACES TO CULTIVATE YOUR #TRIBE

Classes—and that includes exercise

Block and community associations

Places of worship

Local politics

Parents' associations and school activities

Seminars and conferences for work or pleasure

Amateur sports teams, as a player or a coach

Cultural events such as museum openings and concerts

Your neighbors

Support groups

Outdoor associations that organize hiking and kayaking trips

Volunteer activities from hospitals to animal rescue groups

The Internet

Building #Tribes on the Internet

The Internet is one big cluster of #tribes (digital #tribes), constantly forming and breaking apart. A hashtag announces a brand-new #tribe is forming, and soon a community rises. The potential for contact now encompasses the entire world!

This miracle is not without peril. Extreme caution should be used when meeting people on the Internet. It is simply too easy to cover identity and intention in cyberspace. That's not to say you shouldn't, just be careful. Let online friendships grow organically and observe the behavior of others. Is it consistent? Are his or her ideas consistent with your values? If you'd like to meet with the idea of adding them to your #tribe, do. But meet the first few times in a public space where you feel comfortable as you get to know your new acquaintance. Who knows, this might be the best member your #tribe has ever had!

#Tribes and Creating Traditions

My #tribe has many traditions, whether it's preparing a meal together or running toward the lake for that first cool swim of summer. Some of the traditions come from my family and culture and we pass them on to the #tribe. Some come from Kali's side of the #tribe, and those traditions offer wisdom and perspective to our group. Participating in rituals and tradition bonds us to the group. A special cake is baked for every A that comes into the house. Life passages are celebrated with a night out, and everyone is part of the joy. Inclusion. Bonding. Meaning. This is health; this is joyous life.

chapter five

CULTIVATING THE MIND OF THE #HEALTHHERO

B e the still point in a spinning world" could easily be this chapter's title. Nothing in the world will bring you more peace, joy, connection, commitment, understanding, and adventure than believing in something greater than yourself. Belief helps you continue and belief allows you to let go. With a sense of a loving, positive force at work in the world, the #healthhero understands there is no failure, just more learning and life.

Spirituality is an integral part of the #healthhero, just as was true of our four other areas. It is a huge piece of the five components of health, vitality, longevity, and joy. It helps fight depression by taking isolated individuals and connecting them to a greater power: They are not alone. Spirituality also brings other spiritual people together, whether it's in church or in a discussion in a coffee shop, once more reducing isolation in the depressed. Spirituality brings hope, another great gift for the depressed mind. Prayer and meditation dampen the fight-or-flight mechanism and reduce cortisol, the hormone released during stress. Too much cortisol can have negative influences on the immune system, creating ill health, as we've seen with so many of our most prevalent diseases.

Spirituality means many different things to many different people. For some, it is organized religion and involvement with a specific church. For others, it is meditation, yoga, quiet reflection, or private prayer. For still others, it is a walk in nature. As civilization has evolved, many have chosen to take elements of the great world religions—Judaism, Christianity, Islam, Buddhism, and Hinduism—and create their own set of beliefs drawn from some or all. Still others follow the original texts of each religion literally. Native peoples carry beliefs deeply intertwined with the natural world, and their writings prove timely and useful in the struggle to save the environment and the planet.

All faith has a strong impact on health and contributes to creating the #healthhero. Among these five great religions, what are the similarities? That has been an ongoing debate among philosophers, theologians, and religious leaders for century after century.

"I maintain that every religion in the world has similar ideals of love, the same goal of benefiting humanity through spiritual practice, and the same effect of making followers into better human beings. All teach us not to lie or steal or take others' lives, and so on," says His Holiness Tenzin Gyatso, the fourteenth Dalai Lama, in his book, *A Human Approach to World Peace*.

Still others believe that reaching a commonality between religions is impossible because each religion was born to address specific needs. In Islam, you are born without sin. In Christianity, you are born with sin. Imagine how just this point of difference affects the lives of the religions' followers, Peter Donovan pointed out in *Do Different Religions Share Moral Common Ground?* No religion is right or wrong. They are just different, and the more you know about the world religions, the more ideas you have to draw from. Your understanding also contributes a great deal to the ideals of a peaceful world. Part of having a spiritual life is acceptance and respect for those who are different. We are here together!

While some might eschew spirituality, there is ample proof that the human brain is wired for belief. As the brain works over our sensory experiences, it looks for patterns and seeks meaning in those patterns. The more we see and feel that we cannot explain, the deeper our thoughts of something at work greater than ourselves becomes.

Once we believe something, *cognitive dissonance* takes over and we fit our explanations to our beliefs. This is the very bedrock of faith: We trust in something greater than ourselves to guide us. We still trust even if we cannot explain.

Neurologists now speak of the theory of mind. This is the part of the brain that creates a theory of what the other person is thinking and feeling. Author Daniel Goleman brilliantly describes this in his book *Emotional Intelligence.* Theory of mind is the ability to imagine what people feel so you are able to speculate about future actions. Scientists have found the same area of the brain that lights up while discussing spirituality and belief also lights up while formulating a theory of mind. All of this suggests that our most transcendent thoughts and feelings lie exactly where our bonds with others are created. This surely is no coincidence! In 2016, researchers in Utah studied nineteen Mormons and mapped their brain activity. The same areas of the brain lit up during moments the study subjects "felt the spirit" and during periods of intense emotion and reward centers.[1]

I am a fine illustration of theories about bonding and spirituality. Our #tribe was excited and my parents were making the final preparations for a trip; we were going to Tirupati, to visit the Sri Venkateswara Temple in the southeast of India. My mom told me about this amazing spiritual place. Many traveled thousands of miles to visit Tirupati and travel on to the temple, which rested on the Tirumala Hills, 2,800 feet above sea level. My parents had never visited the temple and were equally excited for the trip.

The joy we felt in these simple adventures could not be matched by any technological devices, gadgets, or social media tools. We arrived in Tirupati, a bustling place. Many had traveled far to reach this destination and were anxious to see the temple. However, 2,800 feet of elevation separated us from it! So we began the next phase of our journey, the bus trip up. We roared off to a great start but soon, we were making hairpin turns with a steep drop-off on one side of the road. I was sure that I would not live to see the next day.

To my surprise, we did survive and made it to the top. What a beautiful scene. The temple, built in AD 300, was a huge golden tower, higher than this boy could imagine! There were throngs of people waiting to get into this ancient shrine. We took our place in line and waited patiently. We were tired after a long journey, but our #tribe was together, making the experience delightful. After some time, we reached the entrance, and inside we were amazed at the beauty and presence of the temple. I felt the magnitude of the spiritual trip as I knelt to pray and rejoice in my true joy.

Prayer and spirituality were part of our daily lives. It was clear to me that there was purpose and power greater than me. Although I was cherished as the child of my parents, I was also made aware that I was a part of a universe larger than all of us. My mother, more than anyone else, would teach both my sister and me the importance of spirituality, emphasizing that it played a vital role in our lives every single day. Prayer was twice daily and we all actively participated.

The smell of the puja, or Hindu act of hosting, honor, and worship, was sweet with incense and the variety of beautiful flowers. Spirituality was an important part of our lives, and it was one that we enjoyed. It wasn't a chore that we had to complete but rather a part of who we were as a family, as a #tribe. The pujas invigorated us and kept us grounded. Humility and respect were paramount in our behavior, my parents told us.

They personified these actions. Despite being a world-renowned chemist, my father was grounded and affable. With a great smile, he was warm to both his professional colleagues and to the person who delivered the paper; my #healthhero was dignified, articulate, and empathetic. He knew his considerable worth but never felt the need to broadcast this to the world. The universe and its vastness were clear to him, and he knew his place in it.

My mom is just a breath of fresh air. Warm and personable, she makes friends easily, and to this day, is one of the most empathetic and intuitive people I have ever known. This was clearly derived from her spirituality and her deep belief in prayer and purpose. So I was really given a huge advantage from the time I was born. My family was loving, caring, but also instrumental in helping me cultivate my mind. In India, traditions of spirituality have been present for thousands of years and are not considered an aberration but rather a fundamental part of living.

Moksha, or release from samsara and liberation from karma together with the attainment of nirvana, is a vital concept in the Indian subcontinent, and this understanding of the universe is present in many belief systems on our planet. I was privy to these teachings before the age of seven and have benefited greatly from them. My #healthhero training really began at that time, even though I was unaware of its taking place. I was gaining a strong faith in a mysterious world. In today's technologically driven, stress-infested reality, the ideas of the East are refreshing.

Attempts at the pursuit of spirituality, with practices like meditation, yoga, and prayer, are quite beneficial in attaining a true #healthhero status. The calm this legacy of spiritual learning has given me has allowed me to become who I wanted to become. My purpose is clear to me and my #tribe; we hear our internal compass. We use technology to drive healthy information; technology is not allowed to drive us.

We understand the importance of this awareness in attainment of good health, both spiritually and physically. As we discussed earlier, the #healthhero must be vigilant in purpose, understanding the why, the raison d'être of the journey. Once this happens, you can find the desire and motivation to be the best #healthhero possible. Of course, the #healthhero diet is critical, as is purposeful movement. But this concert of ideas and actions comes full circle with the cultivation of the mind. I learned this at a young age. It's never too late to achieve your goals in spirituality.

YOUR MIND IS CONSTANTLY CHANGING, AND IT'S GREAT!

Neuroplasticity is the general term used for the brain's changing neurochemical pathways. When one part of the brain is damaged, new neurons form, literally "stepping in" to serve the function of the injured area. Activity-dependent plasticity is more of a concern for the #healthhero, both personally and for work with the #tribe. This type of changing of the brain is based on learning and environment.

Just as you can learn to use your left hand instead of your right, eventually changing your DNA and becoming a lefty, you can wire your brain for spiritual practice and growth. The brain's ability to remodel itself for spirituality is the same mechanism that turns off illness-causing DNA and turns on healthy DNA based on what you eat.

For the #healthhero, this spiritual development is critical. Spirituality helps define your purpose and often clarifies your vision. Spirituality operates on its own terms, unseen but infusing all it touches. Practices such as meditation or prayer can help to decrease the "noise," clearing your mind and helping you understand the true meaning of what you want to do and accomplish. When you actually hear your own thoughts, amazing ideas bubble up: new business ideas, solutions to problems, memory and creativity, #tribe activities, and #healthhero thoughts. You make yourself a stronger hero through training the mind and an even stronger hero with the ideas you generate in this calm state. A quiet mind can move mountains. Just ask Martin Luther King Jr. and Gandhi.

We have a prayer room in our house, where we have representations of all the major religions, including Buddhism, Christianity, Islam, Hinduism, and Judaism. We take our kids there and pray daily. We tell them to practice just stopping and taking the time to reflect on the day and be thankful for their gifts. Even our littlest child sits for a few minutes! Our teenage daughter is beginning to benefit from the principles of pausing and reflection. However, the prayer room is not just for the children.

My wife and I are often deep in our thoughts, reflecting on our path and our goals. We want to reach others and persuade them to live healthy lives. Meditation and prayer help us focus and revitalize our minds and our bodies as we prepare for another day of action designed to achieve our goals. Without our spirituality, we would not be successful in achieving these goals. Often we have to regroup and center ourselves, asking the universe for assistance in this pursuit. We place our intentions of education and advocacy in our practice and are rewarded with clarity in thought and action.

Even visitors to our home enter our room of spirituality and are pleasantly surprised at the feelings they experience in their brief encounter with the room. We are open to their beliefs, whether they be devout Christians, Muslims, or even agnostics. Our #tribe's philosophy is that spirituality exists within and outside of religion. We want to be inclusive to the human experience, however it may be expressed.

This practice can then lead to profound changes in mind and body. Folks who are spiritual are healthier and have healthier habits. Research shows that with this practice comes better care of your body, including employing preventive health measures and avoiding harmful behaviors. A ten-year study of a group of Seventh-Day Adventists in the Netherlands yielded some extraordinary findings. As a #tribe, they adopted some sound health ideals such as not drinking, smoking, or consuming pork. But that can only be part of the story, given the results. Within this tightly knit group, men lived 8.9 years longer than average and the women 3.6 years longer. For both men and women, the percentage of dying from cancer decreased dramatically, 60 and 66 percent respectively.

Yes, their healthy lifestyle mattered, but the numbers tell a bigger story: Faith, prayer, support, unconditional love, and hope sent them soaring. Their way of life was literally preventing illness.

What's amazing is that the simple practice of cultivating the mind can actually improve your rates of survival and living a happier, healthier life. In a fascinating study, Giancarlo Lucchetti, MD, PhD, of the Federal University of Juiz de Fora in Brazil, found that having a spiritual life can decrease mortality by 18 percent. Whoa, Nelly! That's fantastic. He found that the power of spirituality was as great as eating fruit and vegetables, and get this: It was as good as taking blood pressure medicines in reducing rates of mortality.

This is powerful, showing the positive health outcomes of cultivating your mind through pausing and reflection. What has been done for thousands of years has now been confirmed by modern measures that we accept and understand. For the #healthhero, this is fantastic—

more tools to add to his or her armamentarium for achieving excellent health.

In Dr. Steven Southwick's work, *Resilience: The Science of Mastering Life's Greatest Challenges*, he writes about how many people overcome tragedies and adversity with the use of religion and spirituality. By searching for purpose in life, these individuals were able to carry on and lead meaningful lives. Difficult situations then became ways to connect with humanity. When we understand that painful circumstances are part of what all of us face, this connects us with others. What was a *Why me?* becomes *I understand that others go through the same challenges and can help.*

These skills are important in dealing with a world that seems to be in perpetual turmoil. From every corner of the globe, there are tragic stories delivered by our news services. We need tools that help ward off the feeling that humanity is crumbling, that we are losing our decency and compassion. I travel the world and can attest to the fact this simply is not true. There are great forces of good at work in the world. Instead of focusing on the latest tragedy or scandal, we should develop empathy and understanding as we shape our worldview through practices that foster spirituality. This attitude attracts other positive attitudes, is viral, and just might save the world.

Stress steals positive feeling. It's difficult to feel anything else when the world is pressing in. It was gloomy and raining when Suresh came to see me. He was dressed well, his suit neatly pressed and his hair perfectly in place. He complained of stomach discomfort and heartburn that woke him several nights a week. His travels took him to the far corners of the planet and he was often not at his best with health concerns. As we continued our conversation, it became clear that Suresh was quite stressed, his face showing the wear of his troubles.

"What else is bothering you?" I asked him. He then told me about his son, who was having difficulties with substance abuse. Despite multiple treatment centers and modes of therapy, Suresh's son was not successful in overcoming his challenges. My patient felt helpless. He was doing everything in his power to advocate for his child but was not finding anything that helped his son. He felt that he was letting his boy down.

Suresh's vital signs were taken and his blood pressure was 170/98. His lab tests showed a high total cholesterol and high LDL (the bad cholesterol) and low HDL (the good cholesterol). I was honest with Suresh. At this rate, he was headed for sure disaster, a heart attack or stroke waiting to happen. Indian men are especially prone to fatal heart attacks! His stress was overwhelming. His work life was fantastic but his family and #tribe were suffering.

I told him that he had to invest time in healing his body with meditation and yoga, as a start. "Don't stop your meds, Suresh," I told him. These would serve as adjuncts, to help his health. I also felt he needed an endoscopy, a test with a lighted scope to look in his gastrointestinal tract. We found damage to his esophagus and his stomach, with ulcerations in both regions. I prescribed a #healthhero diet for him and asked him to follow up in my office.

He returned to me several weeks later; his blood pressure was significantly better. His stomach pain was gone, as were his heartburn symptoms. Initially, yoga was not his favorite activity, but he had learned to love it. He meditated two to three times a week and enjoyed the experience thoroughly. I asked about his son, and although no significant changes had occurred, Suresh's outlook seemed more optimistic!

In his quest to help his son, Suresh was experiencing the great scourge of the twenty-first century. Stress is a killer! It is associated with hypertension and heart disease, and 43 percent of adults are affected with stress. In fact, up to 90 percent of doctor visits are related to stress-induced ailments. Stress and its consequences run rampant in our world today. Its costs are over $300 billion annually in the United States.

Understanding the stress response is important for the #healthhero and his or her goals. Remember, the stress response kept us alive, helping us deal with multiple threats and aggressors through our history. This is the part of the brain that told us to run from an angry woolly mammoth. When you feel stressed, a part of your brain called the hypothalamus sets in motion a series of events that result in your fight-or-flight response, which originates in your lizard brain, a remnant of evolution. Adrenaline and cortisol are released. Adrenaline increases your heart rate and blood pressure and gets your body ready for "battle."

Increased cortisol and increased blood glucose help suppress nonessential parts of your body, like your digestive system. During stressful times of fight or flight, signals are sent to affect your mood and your motivation. These signals have been useful in keeping us alive, letting us have lunch rather than become lunch for a predator during our

Health without peace is short-lived, as internal chaos has a way of breaking the body.

history. However, these responses were meant to be transient, effective for only short periods of time.

With a persistent state of stress, the body's responses I described above are present constantly, affecting your health in a negative manner. Suresh is an example of someone in such a state. His worry was constant, resulting in some of his health concerns. Thus it's very important to find ways to decrease stress levels. The #healthhero's purposeful movement is helpful in decreasing stress, as I described earlier, but spirituality can also be a great tool as well. Putting life's trials and tribulations into perspective and cultivating the mind can really be effective in coping with added stressors.

Meditation is a great way to "quiet" the mind and allow the #healthhero to understand what is really important in his or her life. There are multiple ways to practice meditation. All involve regulating the mind to ease concerns, attain perspective, and improve relaxation. It's also a wonderful way to improve spirituality (you can actually hear your own thoughts!) and is easy to do. It does not require any special equipment and can be done anywhere. The practice of meditation has been around for thousands of years with the first evidence of it occurring in 1500 BC in India. From Buddhist monks to bankers, meditation has been effective in helping us achieve our goals.

THE TWELVE STEPS OF MEDITATION

1. Set your intention. Do you really want to meditate? If the answer is yes, *commit.*

2. Eliminate excuses. From everything. There is no excuse for not meditating, not working out, not supporting your #tribe. Any of it. This is your life. Be in it. Meditation will help you do that.

3. Sit comfortably in a chair or on the floor with legs crossed.

4. Don't get too comfortable. You can't meditate if you keep falling asleep. If this happens, change positions or the temperature in the room. Be alert but calm.

5. Keep a tall spine. Inhale, rolling the shoulders to your ears and exhale lowering them back in place. Whenever you feel yourself getting off balance, do the inhale-exhale shoulder roll.

6. Close your eyes.

7. Maintain a simple breath, in through the nose and out through the nose. Focus on this as your body settles and your nerves calm. Follow your breath in and out in a gentle rhythm.

8. Give it time. You will wiggle and squirm during your initial attempts. It's all a part of learning.

9. Observe without judgment. Let your thoughts come and go without issues of what, why, or when. Just acknowledge the thought and let it go. Return to your breath.

10. Don't go after your thoughts, just let them come to you. Chase nothing. Sit and be. See what comes. Go blank by focusing on your breath again.

11. Shift happens. If you get distracted, don't be overcome with feelings of failure. Distraction is a part of every meditation practice on earth, including those of the great masters.

12. Move if you must. During meditation, legs fall asleep and lips itch. Deal with your issue and go back to following your breath.

Start small by trying 10 minutes and work up to 20, then 30. If this doesn't work for you, don't push it. It may be something you come to at a different phase in life. You might want to try meditating in a different location or at a different time. There are many ways to clear the mind, even meditating while you walk!

Not only does meditation decrease stress and its effects, it has been shown to be useful for our health in general. Dr. Herbert Benson has spent most of his life studying the effect of prayer and meditation on illness and health. Both prayer and meditation evoke the same response: soothing stress and the body and promoting healing. As meditation deepens, the limbic system (it puts emotional "tags" on what is special to us) gets activated. This system controls the nervous system, heart rate, blood pressure, and metabolism, and under the effects of prayer and meditation, the entire organism becomes calm.

PARTHA'S RX

+ Your focus doesn't have to be on God or organized religion, since a belief in anything greater than yourself, including the interconnectedness of life and nature, brings the same health benefits.

+ It's not just that you believe in something, but it is also the repetition of taking time every day to practice it.

+ With the hope and optimism generated by spirituality, people not only have fewer illnesses but also tend to live longer.

+ People who embrace their spirituality are more forgiving than their nonreligious counterparts.

+ Spirituality also offers social support, which is a huge benefit to anyone.

As we learned, spirituality in and of itself is a #healthhero. It helps fight depression by taking formerly isolated individuals and connecting them to a greater power: They are no longer alone. Spirituality also brings other spiritual people together, once more reducing isolation in the depressed. Spirituality brings hope, another great gift for the depressed mind. Prayer and meditation lower the fight-or-flight mechanism and reduce cortisol, the hormone released during stress. As we know, too much cortisol can have negative influences on the immune system, creating ill health.

The last time I felt that great convergence of stress and spirit was on one busy summer day when traffic snarled, as it will, in the Lincoln Tunnel. I was giving a talk and had plenty of time to get to my speech when I landed at the airport in New York City.

The cabdriver wove in and out of traffic in classic New York cabbie fashion, but when we entered the tunnel, everything changed quickly. We came to a dead stop and stayed that way for forty-five minutes. In the beginning I was relaxed, but as the time passed, I became a bit worried that I would be late for the event. I could feel my pulse rate increasing and I felt more anxious. If you've ever been in the Lincoln Tunnel, you would understand my feeling of frustration, as there were no alternatives to get to my destination.

Then something wonderful happened. I began to use my experience in meditation to control my breathing and closed my eyes for a few minutes. I realized that all the people in all the automobiles in this tunnel were suffering the same plight as me. This was just part of the human experience, where all of us face stress and adversity. Within minutes, I was calm again, breathing normally and smiling. I could concentrate on my presentation and how I would tell folks there about the power of meditation.

When I arrived at the event, I was on time and was greeted warmly by the organizers. I went onstage and began the program. During the show, I told the crowd of 4,000 from the New York and New Jersey area about my wonderful experience in the Lincoln Tunnel. I saw smiles in the audience. Many people in that audience dealt with the tunnel and its woes on a daily basis and handled it effectively. Imagine if everyone could treat stress and its effects as we did on that summer day. We would have #healthheroes on every corner of the globe, vanquishing stress and its effects on the mind and body. Cultivating the mind would lead to incredible victories worldwide for all of us!

Meditation is transformational, and luckily for us, there are multiple types. My two favorites are mindfulness meditation and heartfulness. Mindfulness is the practice of becoming aware of the present moment, of both internal and external experiences. This awareness leads to increased spirituality and understanding of oneself. It helps a person become a better listener, with a keener eye for detail. It is one of the most difficult practices that I've attempted, as it requires concentration and dedication. In our multitasking world, being mindful can be challenging, with everyone attempting to achieve more in a given amount of time.

It was June 11, 1997. The NBA finals were in full swing as the Chicago Bulls were taking on the Utah Jazz for the championship. The world's best player, Michael Jordan, was playing for the Bulls, but on this day he was slowed by the flu. It seemed as if the Jazz would handily defeat the Bulls. They had a big lead in the beginning of the game.

Then, to my surprise and that of everyone else in the audience, Jordan slowly came to life. Clearly hampered by his illness, Michael started to make shots and found the energy and strength from within to score 38 points, haul in 7 rebounds, dish out 5 assists, get 3 steals, and perform a block. This particular night has been termed the *flu game*, one of

Jordan's most memorable performances. I remember watching it in amazement.

I didn't know at that time how much of an influence his coach Phil Jackson had on Michael. As an avid basketball fan, I have been amazed by Phil Jackson's success. This legendary coach won eleven championship titles, the most of anyone in the history of the NBA! Jackson used the triangle offense and he had incredible talents such as Michael Jordan, Kobe Bryant, and Shaquille O'Neal, some of the best players ever.

However, Kobe remembers the first time he sat on the floor during practice and meditated! He was sure that George Mumford, who was asked by Jackson to help as a mindfulness expert, was off target. Now Bryant credits Mumford as being one of the most influential people in his sports life. Michael Jordan also used mindfulness training in achieving his amazing results. (It is said that Jordan can meditate for many hours straight!) "Imagine you're a frog on a lily pad," Jackson would say. This mindfulness meditation helped to decrease the stress of competing at an elite level and allowed concentration on the present, not worrying about what has happened or what will happen.

Before all important endeavors—from working with a critically ill patient to giving a talk or working on our health show—I use mindfulness meditation to keep my focus sharp and my mind in the moment. There are multiple challenges, with guest changes, script lineups, and production delays. My mindfulness practice allows me to remain firmly rooted, knowing the purpose of the show is to educate and empower everyone on our planet so we can all be #healthheroes! Helping me to continue on my mission with our television show is wonderful, but mindfulness can do even more in achieving excellent health and wellness of body and spirit.

Heartfulness meditation is another of my favorite types of meditation. Heartfulness has been present for over a hundred years and has a million folks in a hundred countries practicing today. As mindfulness lets you become aware of the present and observe your experience, heartfulness allows you to understand your inner self; it is heart-centered meditation. You focus inward to develop inner strength and peace. As you become more intimate with your inner self, you let go of your worries and your mind calms. With this practice, you become more aware of your true nature and more full of joy and wonder. Taking the time every day to discover your heart center is powerful and can enable you to meet the challenges that every day brings with it.

Spring in the Midwest is a great time for us to rejoice. The winter has finally gone, bringing the warmth and color of the new season while drying up the mud. It was late spring in the Motor City, and the heartfulness summit was taking place in downtown Detroit. I was scheduled to speak there, to discuss the health and wellness benefits of heartfulness. The summit was full of energy and excitement, with thousands in attendance, eager to hear leaders from Google, media companies, and especially the global guide for heartfulness, Kamlesh Patel.

Mr. Patel is a pharmacist by training and has a very successful business in the pharmacy industry. He has practiced heartfulness for decades and travels across the planet speaking about his passion. I was in the front row and was excited to hear him speak. Charming and unassuming, Mr. Patel smiled as he greeted the audience. He told us about the simple nature and benefits of heartfulness. Then he did something wonderful.

"Let's begin a session," he said. He asked us to close our eyes and relax. "Look inside to your heart," he instructed us gently. For the next thirty minutes, we took a journey into our inner selves, with guided meditation by the man himself, Kamlesh Patel! I felt myself going into a state of peace and calm. Thoughts would come and then go as I focused on my heart, my inner self. I was happy, not concentrating on my worries but instead on my soul, my loves, my dreams. It was an incredible experience, one not adequately described by these words.

If I'd had a device on me that day to record my blood pressure and heart rate, I'm sure that both would have been extremely low! It doesn't stop there, however. Your emotional well-being is enhanced, as is your sense of self-worth. Depression and anxiety can be improved because meditation trains your mind to stay in the moment. Meditation shifts thoughts off whatever is creating stress. You can't obsess on the past or future.

Dr. Madhav Goyal at Johns Hopkins University has done a meta-analysis of studies on meditation and depression and anxiety. Remaining in the moment has a beneficial effect and it's typically taught in eight easy sessions. You can meditate almost anywhere at any time: It's all in the way you train your mind.

Your immune system can be strengthened. Meditation produces antibodies that keep foreign invaders from damaging your body; it also stimulates electrical activity in your prefrontal cortex, right anterior insula, and right hippocampus. These are the parts of the brain that control positive emotion, awareness, and anxiety. Arthritis can be lessened, pain levels lowered, and energy levels enhanced! Your emotional well-being and concentration can be significantly improved, with sharpened focus and productivity, a deeply beneficial skill in the ADD world of the Internet. What a great tool for the #healthhero! A simple technique to cultivate the mind leads to unexpected benefits.

After much research, many stops and starts and explorations, I've learned more and more in recent years about different ways to meditate. Whether you create a special space or simply stare at the horizon and clear your mind, all meditation will have a positive impact on the length of your life, the health of your life, and, most important, the state of your mind.

PUTTING IT INTO ACTION

Here are some ideas for meditation that I've used as well as meditation experts and family and friends.

Create a Meditation or "Thinking" Room

Big-screen televisions, computers, and smartphones have created a cacophony of noise throughout the universe. But to find spirituality and peace, you must first quiet the nervous system and the mind. If you can do that, you can tap into and listen to your own wisdom. As you clear the underbrush of unnecessary sound from your mind, a landscape emerges. This is what you believe, what you aspire to, what you dream about. This is you tapping into timeless ideals about life, goodness, purpose, love, and faith in other human beings.

Find a sunny, well-ventilated corner or room in your house. A quiet spot is best. This area can be sparsely decorated—a simple pillow and perhaps a candle—or more elaborately adorned, with statuary, photographs, singing bowls, and gongs. Choose whatever speaks to your spirit.

Wear loose comfortable clothing. Sit cross-legged on a pillow. Turn your gaze inward, practice a slow, gentle yoga breath, and let your mind go blank. As thoughts arise, acknowledge the thought in your mind, then return to blankness. In your mind's eye, visualize a large orange circle on the horizon. Every time your mind wanders from that image, say thank you and return to it. Begin with 5 minutes a day and try to work up to 30. Use guided meditations from apps on your smartphone or join a meditation group to get started.

Quiet contemplation is transformative and has been a tool for great minds for thousands of years, generation after generation. It centers the mind, calms the nervous system, strengthens the immune system, and puts the entire organism (that's you) back into balance. Use this tool. It is completely free, takes only 5 minutes to master, and offers a lifetime of fascinating exploration.

The entire Nandi #tribe uses our meditation corner, including our kids. We encourage them to sit and be quiet for as long as possible. Sure, this is hard for a four-year-old, but our #tribe is being exposed to tools that could very well change their lives.

Breath

The focus of all meditation, awareness of the breath is the cornerstone of stillness.

Simply focus on the air moving into the stomach, up the back, into the back of the throat, and then out slowly. If your attention wanders from your breath, gently turn it back.

Begin with 5 minutes and build up to any amount of time you desire. Use throughout the day as you become stressed.

Kitchen Sink Mindfulness

As you clean the kitchen or do the dishes, focus on your breath and your action. Be aware of the feeling of soap and glass. Notice the temperature of the water as you breathe in and out rhythmically. Clean up after the meal and meditate at the same time!

Candle Meditation

If you have trouble focusing, light a candle and sit in front of it. A flickering candle naturally draws the eye and keeps it. Breathe in and out rhythmically. Increase your time each week just as you would if you weren't using the candle.

Nature Meditation

This is a deeply satisfying meditation, as we are part of the planet. Sit outside on a flat comfortable place, plant the soles of your feet in the grass, and practice breathing. Or go on a walk, focusing on your breath as well as on the sound and color of the natural world.

Visualization

Visualization is the simple technique of closing the eyes and creating a pleasing picture in the mind while breathing in and out. Focus on the image and the breath, and if your mind wanders, gently bring it back to your image.

Prayer or Mantra Meditation

Close your eyes and repeat a mantra or prayer or phrase, focusing on the breath and the words. Repetition has been proven to have positive effects on the brain, calming the entire organism and promoting health and well-being. The more positive the prayer or phrase, the more "change your thoughts, change your life" will be set in motion.

Walking Meditation

The walking meditation should not be confused with the nature meditation. The focus in this form of meditation is on walking with the spine straight and arms swinging by your side, breathing in and out rhythmically. Do this for the course of your daily walk, and exercise and meditation will be rolled into one.

Observer Meditation

While breathing in and out rhythmically, travel outside your body and observe yourself. While this idea may seem odd, it develops self-awareness and insights that help you continue to learn and evolve as a human being. How do you feel looking at yourself meditating? Do you like what you see? Was a series of thoughts negative? How can you adjust that? The #healthhero is always moving toward a wholeness of thought and deed, a consistency, a worldview. Observing yourself is a wonderful tool for shaping the whole human.

Music Meditation

No, this doesn't include reciting all the lyrics to Beyoncé's *Lemonade*. A music meditation requires earphones and soft, unobtrusive music, most often without lyrics. All ambient noise is drowned out, leaving you to focus on the in and out of your breathing as well as on the tune.

Five-Minute Vacation Meditation

Most people have a treasured memory of a beautiful place or moment. If you become stressed during the day, find a spot where you can close your eyes and revisit the place or moment. You'll be refreshed and destressed shortly. Staring at a glorious screen saver and putting yourself in the middle of the scene also works.

Flying Meditation

In your mind, rise fifty feet above the ground and follow a familiar route, making lefts and rights as if you were on foot or in a car. Not only is this good for your memory, you'll be completely immersed in thought during this exercise. When you land, you'll feel rejuvenated and relaxed. Perhaps it's the mental "flying," but I have always found this exercise liberating.

Cloud Meditation

With eyes closed, visualize clouds passing behind your eyelids. Notice the different shapes and colors. Breathe in and out. Visualize more, speeding them up and slowing them down until the end of the meditation. This one is a perfect choice if you are meditating with children or introducing them to the practice.

Meditation on the Sun or the Moon

Many people visualize the horizon and a glowing red orb or shining white ball as they breathe in and out. The ball can rise or stay stationary, it doesn't matter. Keep your attention there, returning your focus to it if your thoughts wander, until the meditation is complete.

Concentric Circle Meditation

Concentric circles are often a symbol of how all of life is connected. This image is a beautiful metaphor for how the spirit interacts with something greater than itself. Simply imagine a rock being thrown into water, focus on the endless rings generated, and continue to breathe quietly and with purpose for the meditation. In a way, this meditation echoes the essence of the #healthhero: five overlapping circles of purpose, nutrition, movement, a sense of belonging through #tribe building, and spirituality. All five areas are constantly in play, creating an overall healthier human being.

Food Meditation

This doubles your lunchtime refreshment. Simply focus on the food as you consume it—its texture, flavor, smell, temperature—and breathe. That's it. Go back to work. This meditation will also help sharpen your senses and deepen your appreciation for being alive. I sometimes do this with a nice piece of dark chocolate—full of antioxidants and pure poetry for the tongue.

Waiting Meditation

Ever find yourself standing in line in the grocery store, staring at another person's basket items? Clear your mind by focusing on your breath and noticing what is around you. Nothing more, nothing less. Don't judge or let feelings of impatience overwhelm you. Continue to breathe and observe calmly. Life is full of waiting, whether in a car or a line, and using the time wisely—remember that the #healthhero integrates the five areas into all facets of life—is a way to achieve your health goals every day.

Body Scan Meditation

The best position for this meditation is lying on your back with your legs extended, arms at your sides. As you breathe in and out, slowly flex and relax your toe muscles. Repeat. Then move your focus to the tops of your feet. Breathe. Become aware of the soles of your feet and slowly travel up the body, focusing on each part, until you reach the crown of your head.

Guided Meditation

All you need for a guided meditation is a teacher or an app download. The app store on your smartphone is full of meditation and mindfulness apps, as is the Internet. Listen with earphones for privacy or find a quiet room. A little search will yield the right guided journey for you. In addition, some meditation apps offer a series of programs that will help you build up to longer and longer meditation sessions.

Not only does this create calm, it will strengthen your ability to focus and concentrate, two mental functions often lost to the ADD of endless screens and stimulation.

Yoga Meditation

The poses and stretching of yoga prepares the body for the meditation to come. If you are a yogi or yogi in training, perform this meditation at the end of your practice, which is hopefully guided by an accredited teacher.

It was a long day of shooting on the set of *Ask Dr. Nandi* and the crew had worked hard the whole day. We were starting a segment of the show focused on yoga, a popular discipline to help with body and mind. The teacher was on set, with a calm smile on her face. Just looking at her gave me a sense of peace. Amid the bustle of television production, she was a breath of fresh air with her steady composure.

As the segment began, I asked her about the benefits of yoga. She answered me with confidence and then the magic started. "Put your hands together and breathe," she said. I complied and after a couple of minutes, the spirit inside me, and the entire studio, was lifted. We were energized, yet calm and content. It was quite interesting to see the body language of the crew. They were equally impressed by the teacher, and many approached her for guidance. That's the power of yoga in the hands of a skilled practitioner.

Yoga has been a tradition of my birth country for thousands of years. Simply put, yoga is a state of being of the body and mind. Physical stances or poses are combined with meditation and controlled breathing exercises. My wife and I practice yoga at home as well as at the studio. As I mentioned earlier, it is quite an effective method to increase the movement of the #healthhero. However, as Kali and I really appreciated, it is a wonderful way to connect with ourselves and others and to relax the mind. This ancient practice dates back to the fifth century BC in India and marries physical activity with spirituality. Yoga has become very popular and accessible to most everyone, making it a great choice for the #healthhero who wants to move with his or her #tribe while cultivating the mind.

Yoga is safe for most folks and works with the limitations of your body and health. Your doctor should guide you in understanding if it's safe for you. There are many types of yoga. Some popular types are:

Hatha. This combines movement with controlled breathing. This is the type of yoga most people associate with the word.

Iyengar. Here blocks, straps, and chairs are employed to help you move your body into the proper alignment.

Bikram. This is also called hot yoga, because the poses are done in a heated room.

Vinyasa. This form of yoga uses poses that flow into one another.

Power Yoga. A higher intensity practice that builds muscle and is faster paced for aerobic benefit.

Ashtanga. A specific series of poses, combined with a special breathing technique.

If yoga and meditation don't work for you, here are some ideas to clear the head from a different direction. All are effective and closer to things you actually do day to day. This way, you simply layer the meditation atop and voilà!

Spiritual Exercises

Like all parts of a human being, spirituality needs to be used, like a muscle, to develop and grow stronger. This is a workout for your soul, if you will. You might be highly religious and working your spirit through the prayer and traditions of that faith. You might have a more personalized form of spirituality, a form that can take elements of many religions and is specific to you. All that is required is a belief in something larger than you, some force that binds all living things together.

Read

Spend 15 to 30 minutes a day reading about spirituality. If you grew up in a religious tradition, simply extend the time spent studying the texts of your faith. If your spirituality is just taking shape, try an overview of the world's religions and be aware of how you feel when you read about each. Notice if you are drawn to certain ideas more than others. Explore the spiritual writings of native peoples, especially important in our relationship to nature and the Earth.

Attend a Religious Service

If you do not participate in organized religion, give it a chance. Ask one of your family, friends, or neighbors who regularly attend to allow you to join them. Pay close attention to what is said and done and to how you feel about it. Contemplate what you've heard and whether you'd like to hear more. Did you like the sense of community? Do you want to be a part of it?

Attend a Service Outside Your Religion

Some of the most moving and thought-provoking moments emerge when you allow the ways of another spiritual tradition to enter your heart and mind. You see differences and profound similarities. You gain understanding about cultures, history, and worldviews. Most important, human faces emerge, unique and hopeful, just like yours.

Socratic Spirituality, or the Art of Inquiry

Socrates was a classical Greek philosopher who lived from 470–469 BC to 399 BC. Little is known about him except through the writings of others—in particular, Plato. Socrates gave the world the Socratic method, a way of questioning to isolate and provide insight into whatever issue is before you. (The Socratic method is an ancient philosophy at work in all our lives to this day. Our legal system is built upon it and it's useful in many endeavors, from editing a book to figuring out who ate your pint of ice cream while you were at work.) Contemplate your ideas about spirituality as a series of questions, each leading to the next. Start with "What do I believe? Why?" and then ask yourself the next question and the next as they enter your mind.

Forgiveness Exercise

From soaring cathedrals to twelve-step meetings, *forgiveness* is a word that rings out over and over. The ability to forgive is an essential component of spirituality and the joyful life. If you hold on to negative thoughts about people or situations, detox. Gather small rocks or pebbles for as many people as you need to forgive or as many situations as you need to let go of. Sit down beside any water you can find—stream, pond, ocean, or even bathtub. Pick up a stone, hold it tightly, and think about the perceived or real hurt. Understand that it is past. What did you learn? Understand that it cannot hurt you again. How can you use the experience in the future? Throw the rock into the water and as it sinks, let go.

Serve for an Hour a Week

If spirituality is acknowledging the connection of all living things, what higher honor can you give than by helping other living things? Providing for your family and helping friends is of course a part of this exercise. But to really use this muscle, try stretching it toward those you do not know, those who do not have your resources. Set aside one hour a week for service. It may mean climbing out of bed early on a weekend, but do it. The rewards are massive. Read to children, serve food to the homeless, work at a food pantry, or tutor. So many could use your skills; you are wanted and needed.

Contemplation

The image of a brown-robed monk in a mountaintop cave comes to mind with the word *contemplation*. But contemplation should be part of daily life for everyone. It is a way to check in with your own spirit, lower the noise, and see how you feel about what is happening within and around you. Sit in a chair, feet flat on the floor, relax, and close your eyes. Replay events through your spirit, noting how scenes and situations made you feel.

Did you respond in a way you were proud of? How could you do better? Did you give offense? Spend 5 to 10 minutes at first, building up to a half hour.

Share Ideas

Some consider spirituality a highly personal subject. Most enjoy and learn from lively discussion and the sharing of ideas about faith, religious texts, and service. What everyone believes is not the core issue; the sharing is. Join a study group for any religious text. Attend a secular class on the world's religions at a local university. (Classes are now available online, with interactive capabilities for the discussion part.)

You could also form a more casual once-a-month evening for discussions with friends. Pay close attention to how people use what they learn in their day-to-day lives.

Circle of Three

Among all the people you know, how many different religions do they follow? Find two others, not of your own faith, and start a breakfast or lunch club. Talk about your differences. Talk about your similarities. Learn about their families, their histories, and their cultures. Cook for each other and tell stories. This will deepen your understanding and respect for other religions as well as work that most important of spiritual muscles, empathy.

Pray or Repeat a Mantra or Poem

All three of these activities are repetitive and light up the front part of the brain, the language center. Recitation stabilizes neural pathways, creating a calmness of mind and spirit. Sit in a comfortable chair, feet flat on the ground, eyes closed. Recite a favorite prayer, mantra, or poem stanza over and over in your mind for 3 to 5 minutes. Try this mind-calming technique before going into a deeper contemplation.

Thought Watching

Negativity is kryptonite for the growth of spirit. With this in mind, spend a few minutes of contemplation going over the thoughts, words, and deeds of the day. What are you feeling negative about? Is there anyone you are holding back or vice versa with negative words? What do you believe about yourself? Is it negative? How can you change this? Thought watching is simply an awareness of your own thought patterns and the way you can reach the best possible life.

Empathy Exercise

Empathy is when you understand how the person born in the bed next to you feels. Or at least you believe you do, based on your own experience or what you've seen. Empathy is the ability to put yourself in another person's shoes, enabling you to feel connected to other living beings. Our spirit pulls at us to offer help, hope. This spirit muscle can be exercised like any other, the more frequently the better. Since watching and listening are the cornerstones of empathy, that's what this exercise requires. Every night before you go to sleep, recall a story someone told you in the course of the day. Think about how that person might have felt about the story. Bring the story up the next time you see him or her. Let that person know the story was heard. He or she was heard.

Gratitude Exercise

It's as simple as this: Wherever you are, when your head hits the pillow, spend your last waking moments thinking about the things in your life you are grateful for. Some of the items on your list will remain constant, like your family, and the rest could change. Notice if they do and in what way. Never stop being grateful and express it when appropriate.

Natural World Contemplation

Nothing leaves us more in awe than a beautiful sunset or a snow-covered mountain. Yet how often in the hustle and bustle of an increasingly urban life do we make an effort to appreciate and connect to the natural world? Sit in a park at lunch and watch a ladybug. On a weekend, go hiking in the nearest woods. Sit. Close your eyes. Inhale the air deeply. Exhale. Repeat. Then open your eyes and take in all the detail of what is before you, contemplate how it works together, the grand design of it all.

Art Therapy

Art has long been used to help both the creator and the observer access emotions, so put some art into your life. Go to an art museum with the intention of finding a beautiful work that moves you. Observe both it and yourself carefully. What do you feel? Why do you feel it? What speaks to you most? The same experience is available at a concert, where music, believed to be a primal form of communication, triggers thoughts and emotions. Notice how you feel. It's all a part of figuring out what moves you, what opens you up to greater ideas and deeper thought and feeling.

Yoga

Whatever style is your favorite, yoga has marvelous health effects. It can help with stress reduction and improve well-being. Instructors often talk about "taking yoga off the mat." This refers to transferring the strength of the body and mind from your yoga practice into your life, dealing with the obstacles of daily life. You can improve arthritis and reduce the risk factors of chronic disease, such as depression and heart disease. As I spoke about previously, the movement of the #healthhero is optimized, leading to increased fitness.

Yoga's strengthening of the mind is critical for the #healthhero in achieving his or her goals. While we spoke of yoga in chapter 3, which included poses you could do anywhere, I've added a few more here. These poses are more conducive to deep contemplation than others I've found. You may find different poses work better for you during meditative exercises.

Yoga Breathing

Again, this can be done at your desk, in the middle of a staff meeting, or on a train, bus, or plane. Sit or stand with your feet firmly planted on the ground. Inhale, pulling the air into your abdomen and feeling it expand. Pull the air up all the way into your chest. Then exhale slowly, contracting the abdomen and feeling it draw in. Repeat until you feel calmer and more centered. You should breathe in this manner throughout every meditation. Your blood will get more oxygen and your heart rate will stabilize.

Child's Pose

One of the most relaxing poses in yoga, this is a perfect way to stretch out and calm your nervous system before bed. Kneel on the edge of a thick towel, blanket, or mat. Sit back on your knees, lower your head to the floor, and stretch your arms out in front of you. Take 5 deep yoga breaths in this position. Sleep like a baby.

Drawing-in-Senses Pose

Sit in a chair or on the floor. Remove your eyeglasses if you wear them. Put your hands in front of your eyes, with your palms turned toward your face, the tips of your middle fingers touching your eyes. Closing your eyes, place your middle fingers very gently along your eyelids, the tips of the fingers touching the inner corners of your eyes. Place the index fingers along the line of your eyebrows, rest your ring fingers on the corners of your nostrils, and rest your pinkies on your upper lips or at the corners of your mouth. Finally, close the flaps of your ears with your thumbs.

Let your eyes, ears, nose, and tongue become completely relaxed. Journey inside for 5 to 10 minutes. Each week, add a little time to this pose, working toward a silent 15- to 20-minute trip into your spirit.

Legs-up-the-Wall Meditation

I've combined a well-known yoga pose that requires no physical effort with simple deep breathing for this meditation. Place the base of your spine against where the floor meets the wall and rotate your legs straight up the wall. You'll feel a stretch running down your hamstrings. Breathe deeply. In addition to the calming benefit of the gentle rise and fall of your lungs and belly, the pose relieves tired leg muscles, reduces edema in legs and feet, gives you the benefits of inversion without the physical effort or safety issues, calms the nervous system, and quiets the mind.

Turn your focus within. Listen to the sound of your breath as it enters and leaves your body. Let go of concerns about your work, your day, your life.

Let yourself linger here as long as you are comfortable. When you release your legs to the floor, sit with your eyes closed for a few more moments, letting the peace of your inner self come with you, back to the outer world.

Savasana, or Corpse Pose

How can something with such an alarming name be so good for you? Savasana is perhaps the most important pose in all of yoga, but most

Western classes spend only a short time in the pose at the end of the practice. Traditionally, savasana is held much longer at the end of practice and is a cornerstone of yoga, ground zero for the power of calm.

The "corpse" reference has to do with the position of the body. You should be flat on your back, completely comfortable on a mat or blanket, with arms and legs stretched out in four directions at 45-degree angles. Your eyes are closed. Focus on each breath moving in and out of your body. Scan the body for any physical discomfort, flexing and slightly moving areas of tightness or pain. The asana—breath—is released, deepening it and slowly releasing control of the mind and body. Deep relaxation and rejuvenation take place.

At the end of your savasana, roll on your side, bringing your legs up into a fetal position. Remain there for a short while before rising.

The benefits of this meditative pose astonish: heart rate and respiration decrease and calm; blood pressure drops; muscles release tension; there is a reduction in anxiety; and focus, concentration, productivity, and memory are all improved.

Never is the advocacy of the #healthhero more important than now. By cultivating the mind, achieving spirituality and inner strength, the #healthhero can prevail in his or her advocacy. The #healthhero can fight for loved ones when no one else seems to care, listen, and understand. Health-care decisions are being taken out of the hands of our physicians, and the lack of continuity in care leads to strangers as caregivers, adding to the chances of error and a disturbing lack of empathy and advocacy. What was once a given—that your health-care provider will act as your champion—is no longer true. We all need the spirit, the heart, and the mind of the #healthhero to champion the needs of our #tribe members.

The strength of our minds and souls helped us to do something that really helped our #tribe: forgiveness. You may ask yourselves, "How could you forgive someone who wronged your father? How can you forgive caregivers who did not care if he lived or died?"

Well, forgiveness is a difficult concept. By forgiveness, I don't mean that we excuse those who wronged my biggest hero. Rather, it refers to letting go of the blame and negative thoughts. These negative thoughts can often be paralyzing to you, the victim. By releasing these thoughts, I was able to move forward with my #tribe and help my father. This tradition of forgiveness is common in major religions from Buddhism and Christianity to Islam and Judaism.

Besides helping you strengthen your mind, forgiveness can be used to reduce feelings of anger and hurt. Your blood pressure, immune system, and heart health are also improved. This is a great technique for the #healthhero to master. Forgiveness can be a revolutionary tool in achieving inner strength and peace.

Fear is a strong emotion. It allows many a #healthhero to fail. Fear doesn't let us function optimally. Why is fear such a strong emotion? Through history, fear has been instrumental in keeping us alive. But many events and objects that are fear-inducing are not life-threatening, and this fear blocks us from bonding with others, giving and receiving support, and taking on a new challenge. Fear can be a good indicator of growth in a person, provided he or she pushes through it and takes on the challenge anyway. Fear tells you there might be a risk so you can assess it and proceed accordingly. Don't hate fear, but don't let it get a grip.

———————

I was gasping for breath as I stepped out of the shallow pool. Several small children were giggling at me, a six-foot-two man frightened in four feet of water. They couldn't believe it. It was obvious to me. I was taking swimming lessons as an adult, having never learned the skill as a child. My bout with rheumatic fever as a child kept me from learning how to swim. I wanted to be a resource for my children when they were in the water, so here I was, ready to take the proverbial plunge into the water that I feared.

When I entered the water, my fear took over completely and I was sure that I would drown. This fear was of course irrational given my height, but it felt very real for me. My heart was pounding and I was positive that I would drown. Then I used my techniques of meditation and breathing to relieve these fears. Slowly but surely, I became more confident, using the mind of the #healthhero to conquer this obstacle. My patient swim instructor was amazing, helping me succeed in my quest.

On our show, *Ask Dr. Nandi*, Dr. Rick Hanson appeared as a guest and stated, "Throughout time, we as humans have strived to eat lunch and not *be* lunch." Our fear, when used properly, has helped us to succeed and thrive. Though in modern times, our threats don't typically come from predators trying to do us harm.

Instead, they come from a negative comment, an expression of discontent or rejection from a partner. Financial concerns stir fear. News reports bring war into the living room. These stimuli set off the same triggers that our ancestors felt. Fight, flight, or freeze begins. The #healthhero can achieve success in his or her quest at achieving good health and wellness by understanding and mastering fear. Imagine *not* being afraid to fail, *not* being afraid that the person across from you is hostile. This mastery of fear will break the cycle of fight, flight, or freeze. It will allow the #healthhero to work optimally, not paralyzed by the ancient concepts instilled in us so long ago.

Now the #healthhero can go confidently, armed with the knowledge of great nutritional tools, effective techniques of movement, the power of the #tribe, and the mature cultivation of the mind. Through building a strong body, mind, and spirit, the #healthhero can meet whatever difficulty life presents. As advocates for themselves and their health and well-being, as well as advocates for their #tribe, #healthheroes can use their tools with ease, cape flying, helping our planet achieve better health, longevity, and joyful living.

Health is about what you put in your mouth and what you put in your mind. Whole foods and positive thoughts are our mantra! Remember that. Preventive medicine, shining health and well-being, are all inside you, waiting to be explored. You can change at any time, and regardless of your lifestyle, it's never too late to get back on track. Nature recovers, you recover. That is part of the wonder of being alive.

Human beings are both fragile and strong, easily wounded and resilient. A contradiction, sure, but if we could harness the great and sometimes mysterious powers within us all, what would the world look like? Vibrant health, respect, serenity, and understanding are inside of you, and the more you develop these muscles, the more fulfilled you will be.

Hopefully, your #tribe will include many #healthheroes, and together you can build your community. A sense of belonging develops and you will find your life becoming larger, more open, more exciting and full of possibility. You'll find new ideas, get support, and have company when you do what you love to do. Bond and build, that's what the #healthhero does, and I feel that anyone who has read this book is completely ready to join the #tribe I have built.

My #tribe welcomes you. We are so happy you are here, a new #healthhero, helping yourself and the world to heal, grow strong, and be great.

Namaste indeed.

ACKNOWLEDGMENTS

To my wife and life partner, Kali, thank you for being my everything. Your dedication, support, and unwavering love were instrumental in helping define my purpose and life's work.

To my original heroes, my mother and father, Ruby and Uma, whose leadership, courage, and empathy shaped my life. Thank you for making me who I am today.

To my sister, Mohua, thank you for your encouragement, support, and love. I have learned so much from your selflessness and devotion.

To my children, Partha, Shaan, and Charley: Thank you for helping me understand the meaning of true love and happiness. You are my world!

To my literary agent, Lisa Hagan, thank you for your support and advocacy. You rock!

To my editor, Beth Wareham, you are a magician and a visionary! Thanks for everything.

To Michele Martin, my editor at North Star Way, I love your enthusiasm, sage advice, and wisdom. Thanks for your leadership.

To Cindy Ratzlaff at North Star Way, thank you for always asking the right questions and encouraging me to push the limits.

To Diana Ventimiglia, my editor at North Star Way, I love your style and your soul. Thanks for all you do.

To Mr. Glover, my beloved teacher at Centennial High School, thank you for your guidance, encouragement, and leadership. You gave me the tools I needed to help me reach my goals.

To Mahatma Gandhi, whose teachings and work inspire me every day. Namaste, sir!

To my team at Ask Dr. Nandi: Darcie Purcell, Lora Probert, Marjorie "Jo" McAllister, and Greg Gnyp, thanks for your amazing work and support. I couldn't have done it without you.

NOTES

introduction

1 Diener, Ed, University of Illinois and Chan, Micaela, University of Texas at Dallas, *Applied Psychology: Health and Well-Being* © 2011 The International Association of Applied Psychology.

2 Cohen, Randy MD, MS, Bavishi, Chirag MD, MPH, Rozanski, Alan MD, *Psychosomatic Medicine*, vol. 78, no. 2 (February/March 2016): 122–33, doi:10.1097/PSY.0000000000000274 Systematic Review/Meta-Analysis.

chapter one

1 Hamblin, James, "Health Tip: Find Purpose in Life," the *Atlantic* (November 3, 2014): https://www.theatlantic.com/health/archive/2014/11/live-on-purpose/382252/.

2 Tan, Erwin, Associate Professor, Johns Hopkins Center on Aging and Health, John Hopkins University, et al, *Journals of Gerontology*, vol. 63, no. 1 (January 2008).

3 Hill, Patrick and Turiano, Nicholas, University of Rochester, Association for Psychological Science (May 8, 2014). http://journals.sagepub.com/doi/abs/10.1177/0956797614531799.

4 Putnam, R. D. E Pluribus Unum: Diversity and Community in the 21st Century: The 2006 Johan Skytte Prize Lecture. *Scandinavian Political Studies* [Internet]. 2007;30 (June 2007): 137–74.

chapter three

1 *Arch Intern Med.* (2010);170(4): 321–31. doi:10.1001/archin ternmed.2009.530.

2 Steven C. Moore, PhD, MPH, et al, *JAMA Intern Med.* (2016); 176(6): 816–25: doi:10.1001/jamainternmed.2016.1548.

chapter four

1 Berkman, L. F., Syme, S. L., et al. *American Journal of Epidemiol.* (Feb 1979): 109(2): 186–204.

chapter five

1 Ferguson, Michael, et al., University of Utah, http://dx.doi.org/10 .1080/17470919.2016.1257437

RESOURCES

Here are some additional ideas for research to get you started on a #healthhero path:

chapter one: Find Your Purpose

Sign up for Healthhero Magazine: http://askdrnandi.com/health hero-magazine/

Take a quiz and find your bliss: http://thinksimplenow.com/happiness/life-on-purpose-15-questions-to-discover-your-personal-mission/

Unexpected ways to find your purpose: http://www.huffingtonpost.com/shannon-kaiser/3-unexpected-ways-to-find_b_5176511.html

How to read 3 signs telling you your purpose in life: https://www.entrepreneur.com/article/247433

Wiki how to find purpose in life: http://www.wikihow.com/Find-Your-Purpose-in-Life

How to find your purpose and become a better person: http://www.lifehack.org/articles/lifestyle/how-find-your-lifes-purpose-and-make-yourself-better-person.html

Medical heroes: https://quizlet.com/5854285/famous-medical-heroes-flash-cards/

Helping you to find your life purpose: https://www.psychology today.com/blog/prescriptions-life/201311/helping-you-find-your-life-purpose

How to find your life purpose: https://zenhabits.net/life-purpose/

Find purpose when your life is crashing into chaos: http://tinybuddha.com/blog/3-steps-to-find-your-purpose-when-life-is-crashing-into-chaos/

Book Recommendations for Finding Purpose:

The Purpose Driven Life by Rick Warren

The Gifts of Imperfection by Brené Brown, PhD, LMSW

Mountains Beyond Mountains by Tracy Kidder

A New Earth: Awakening to Your Life's Purpose by Eckhart Tolle

Write It Down, Make It Happen by Henriette Anne Klauser

Focus: The Hidden Driver of Excellence by Daniel Goleman

On the Shortness of Life: Life Is Long if You Know How to Use It by Seneca

Man's Search for Meaning by Viktor E. Frankl

Do What You Love, the Money Will Follow by Marsha Sinetar

What Do You Want to Do Before You Die? by The Buried Life

Act Locally Through National Organizations:

VolunteerMatch.org

HealthCareVolunteer.com

Corporation for National and Community Service

GoEco.org

Save Our Seas Foundation

Nature.org

ChristianVolunteering.org

JewishVolunteer.com

IslamicReliefUSA.org

Habitat.org

MakeItRight.org

WorldTeach.org

VolunteerAlliance.org

chapter two: The #HealthHero Nutrition Plan

Here are some of our go-to websites for healthy eating ideas and resources:

AskDrNandi.com—healthy cooking recipes: http://askdrnandi .com/cooking-with-dr-nandi/

WebMD.com—healthy eating guidelines: http://www.webmd .com/women/guide/nutrition-101-how-to-eat-healthy#1

CookingLight.com—reduced calorie and whole food recipes: http:// www.cookinglight.com

NutritionFacts.org—calorie and nutritional makeup of foods: nutritionfacts.org

MyFitnessPal.com—calorie and nutritional make-up of foods: www .myfitnesspal.com/food/calorie-chart-nutrition-facts

EatRight.org—latest trends impacting food supply and more: www .eatright.org/resource/food/nutrition/nutrition-facts-and-food-la bels/the-basics-of-the-nutrition-facts-panel

NutritionData.self.com—nutritional information and recipes: nutritiondata.self.com

EatingWell.com—healthy recipes: www.eatingwell.com/recipes/ 18410/low-calorie/quick-easy/

Health.Harvard.edu—Dr. Walter Willett's healthy eating plate: www.health.harvard.edu/healthy-eating-plate

NIH vitamin and minerals resource: https://ods.od.nih.gov/fact sheets/list-VitaminsMinerals/

Book Recommendations for Nutrition, Cooking, and Eating:

How Not to Die by Michael Greger, MD, and Gene Stone

Thug Kitchen by Thug Kitchen

The Complete Vegetarian Cookbook by America's Test Kitchen

Eat Fat, Get Thin by Mark Hyman, MD

The China Study by T. Colin Campbell, PhD, and Thomas M. Campbell II, MD

Eat, Drink, and Be Healthy by Walter Willett, MD

Prevent and Reverse Heart Disease by Caldwell B. Esselstyn Jr., MD

The Essential Diabetes Book by The Mayo Clinic

Anticancer: A New Way of Life by David Servan-Schreiber, MD, PhD

The Whole30 by Melissa Hartwig and Dallas Hartwig

Cooking, Recipes, and Healthy Eating Apps:

Allrecipes Dinner Spinner by All Recipes, Inc.

Food Network in the Kitchen by Television Food Network

100 Healthy Recipes with 3 Ingredients by Dusan Grujin

Fit Men Cook—Healthy Recipes by Nibble Apps Ltd.

BigOven by BigOven.com

Yummly by Yummly

Weber's On the Grill by Weber-Stephen Products LLC

Tender—Social Food by Omnomicon LLC

SideChef: Step-by-step cooking by SideChef

NYT Cooking by The New York Times Company

Grocery and Meal Delivery Services:

The Internet brings great food to your doorstep in the form of fresh ingredients or the specific components for a fresh meal. If you don't have time to shop and prep, it's worth exploring.

Instacart: Enter your zip code and the groceries arrive in an hour. Could it be this easy? It could. Make the Internet work for your life.

Whole Foods: Enter your order online and swing by on the way home to pick it up, trimming angst—and time—off the end of your day.

AmazonFresh: A fee is required to join and then you'll get your fresh ingredients within the day.

HelloFresh: Currently in 30 states, these meals are designed by two renowned chefs—from Momofuku and Eleven Madison Park in New York City—and arrive with the ingredients ready to go.

Blue Apron: Dedicated to sustainable farming practices and fresh ingredients, you'll receive your meal already prepped. You follow the recipe and add heat. Do the math: It could be a cost saver for you.

chapter three: The #HealthHero Movement Plan

Helpful websites featuring exercises and workouts:

Bodybuilding.com

Yoga.com

YogaJournal.com

PilatesAnytime.com

MensHealth.com Interval Training

Cycling Videos Online

Barre3.com Barre Workout

JessicaSmithTV.com walking workouts

Coolrunning.com

DailyBurn.com

TrainOnline.com

Books on Movement:

The Yoga Bible by Christina Brown

Yoga Anatomy by Leslie Kaminoff and Amy Matthews

The New Encyclopedia of Modern Bodybuilding by Arnold Schwarzenegger

The Women's Health Big Book of Pilates by Brooke Siler

Pilates Anatomy by Rael Isacowitz and Karen Clippinger

Bigger Leaner Stronger by Michael Matthews

The Running Revolution by Dr. Nicholas Romanov and Kurt Brungardt

Wild by Cheryl Strayed

A Walk in the Woods by Bill Bryson

BodyMinder: Workout and Exercise Journal by F. E. Wilkins

Fitness Apps for Smartphones:

Stepz: Set a step goal every day and this app will tell you when you reach it, and it includes a calorie count.

Health Data: Now on iPhones, you can use this as a good overview of your daily exercise and track your progress. This serves as a log or journal and includes how to track body changes.

Fitness Buddy: The app has every exercise categorized by body part, equipment requirements, and difficulty. You can also track your progress and check if you are overtraining.

Nike+ Training Club: This app keeps you from ever getting bored with exercise in over 130 workouts for all levels.

Map My Run—GPS Running and Workout Training by Under Armour: Using GPS, you can map your routes based on training levels and hit the road, tracking calorie burns and progress as you add length and difficulty.

Map My Walk—GPS Walking and Step Training by Under Armour: See above, only for walking, a great exercise!

Peloton Cycle—Live: Live stream a spinning class on any stationary bike wherever you are. Just bring your smartphone and a pair of ear buds.

Down Dog—Great Yoga Anywhere: Brand-new vinyasa yoga sequences anywhere, anytime.

Pilates—Lumowell: This app will teach you the exercises, build your routines for you and track your progress.

MotionTraxx—Workouts Treadmill by Motion Traxx: Learn how to use your treadmill time in ways you never expected, including integrating free weights and interval training to strengthen and burn fat.

chapter four: The #HealthHero #Tribe

The Internet is nothing more than a big hive of communication waiting to connect one to another. Check out these websites:

Nextdoor.com: This site allows you to share thoughts on where to eat, what to do, crime notices, local concerts and theater, rallies, and more. Get to know your neighbors and see if a #tribe grows.

Meettheneighbors.org: Less elaborate than Nextdoor, this app allows you to set up a time, date, and place to meet neighbors. It's a great first start.

Meetup: This is where you can find every passion on earth and a group that enjoys meeting and talking about it. You only sign up here. To socialize, you have to go to the meet ups.

Active.com: Here is the perfect spot for sports and outdoor lovers. It will provide information about events, contests, teams, and groups in your area.

Books About #Tribe and Belonging:

The Blue Zones by Dan Buettner

Thrive: Finding Happiness the Blue Zones Way by Dan Buettner

The Little Book of Hygge: Danish Secrets to Happy Living by Meik Wiking

Tribe by Sebastian Junger

How to Win Friends & Influence People by Dale Carnegie

Hanging Out, Messing Around, and Geeking Out by Mizuko Ito and Sonja Baumer

Love & Survival: The Healing Power of Intimacy by Dean Ornish, MD

The New Breed: Understanding and Equipping the 21st Century Volunteer by Jonathan McKee and Thomas W. McKee

Volunteer: A Traveller's Guide to Making a Difference Around the World by Lonely Planet

The Undoing Project: A Friendship That Changed Our Minds by Michael Lewis

chapter five: Cultivating the Mind of the #HealthHero

These websites offer reference and how-to insight into stress reduction, meditation, and contemplation:

Lumosity.com: You'll work on your critical and executive capabilities as well as your memory.

FreeMeditations.com: This site has everything from guided meditations from Descartes to the Buddhist meditation.

Breathing exercises/YouTube.com: YouTube is a rich playground for finding how-to videos for exercise, yoga, meditation, and more.

BarrattBreathInstitute.com: You can take online classes in breath work to increase energy and decrease anxiety so you thrive.

Marc.UCLA.edu: Here are free guided meditations for anything from loving-kindness to sleep preparation, all in English and Spanish.

YogaJournal.com/meditationposes: This short rundown takes you through all the ways to sit, stand, lie down, or move through your meditation.

Meditations/YouTube.com: The choice of guided meditations is vast. Find the ones that suit your needs.

Mindful.org: This large site teaches and helps develop the practice of mindfulness for decreased stress and increased focus and calm.

SharonSalzberg.com: For all things loving-kindness meditation, look to Sharon.

MayoClinic.org/stretching: Detangling muscles and sinews has an enormously relaxing effect on the body. And injury rates go down.

Apps to Cultivate the Mind:

Headspace: Surrender 10 minutes of your day to this trainer for your mind. You can track progress and motivate friends as well.

The Mindfulness App: Here's a meditation app that reminds you it's almost time to meditate.

Buddhify: This app presents meditations to help solve specific problems such as "travel," "going to sleep," or "walking in the city."

Buddhify2: This version is geared to the urban dweller.

Omvana: This is simply the largest collection of meditations available in any app on the market.

Meditation Timer: Once you start flying on your own and don't want the voice in your ear, you'll need this app to tell you when to touch back down.

Breathe2Relax: Breath belongs with mind because a well-oxygenated, relaxed brain is a brain functionally at its best.

Simply Being: This beloved app is one of the best for both beginners and the more experienced. You choose background and music.

Equanimity: This is the best of the best, an app that includes the meditations, journal, timer, badge and icon reminders, and other ways to keep you on track.

Calm: An app with beautiful sounds and images that is suitable for beginners to experts.

Books to Cultivate the Mind:

Thinking, Fast and Slow by Daniel Kahneman

Emotional Intelligence by Daniel Goleman

The Varieties of Religious Experience by William James

The Miracle of Mindfulness by Thich Nhat Hanh

Lovingkindness by Sharon Salzberg and Jon Kabat-Zinn

The Alchemist by Paulo Coelho

The Relaxation Response by Herbert Benson, MD, and Miriam Z. Klipper

Buddha in Blue Jeans by Tai Sheridan

Thrive by Arianna Huffington

The Brain's Way of Healing by Norman Doidge, MD

Books on the Mind, Spirituality, Stress, Mood, and Relaxation:

Declutter Your Mind by S. J. Scott and Barrie Davenport